Customized Healing

Blending the Best of Eastern and Western Medicine

Mark Mincolla, Ph.D.

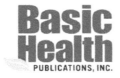

Basic Health PUBLICATIONS, INC.

The information contained in this book is based upon the research and personal and professional experiences of the author. It is not intended as a substitute for consulting with your physician or other healthcare provider. Any attempt to diagnose and treat an illness should be done under the direction of a healthcare professional.

The publisher does not advocate the use of any particular healthcare protocol but believes the information in this book should be available to the public. The publisher and author are not responsible for any adverse effects or consequences resulting from the use of the suggestions, preparations, or procedures discussed in this book. Should the reader have any questions concerning the appropriateness of any procedures or preparation mentioned, the author and the publisher strongly suggest consulting a professional healthcare advisor.

Basic Health Publications, Inc.
www.basichealthpub.com

Library of Congress Cataloging-in-Publication Data

Mincolla, Mark Dana.
    Customized healing : blending the best of Eastern and Western medicine / Mark Mincolla.
        p. cm.
    Includes bibliographical references and index.
    ISBN 978-1-59120-298-1 (Pbk.)
    ISBN 978-1-68162-707-6 (Hardcover)

    1. Medicine, Chinese—Popular works. 2. Nutrition—Popular works. I. Title.
    R601.M52   2011
    610—dc23

                                                        2011044732

Editor: Roberta W. Waddell
Typesetting/Book design: Gary A. Rosenberg
Cover design: Mike Stromberg

Contents

PART 3   The Contemporary West

I would like to dedicate this book to the Tao

There is an increasing sense that certain ancient and esoteric healing practices, long ignored by Western science, may in fact represent profound insights into the very nature of healing.

In Western society, health is defined in strictly clinical terms by physicians. In Eastern societies, sickness is disruption, imbalance, and the manifestation of malevolent forces in the flesh. Health and healing represent a state of balance, of harmony, and for most of these societies it is something holy.

—WADE DAVIS, PH.D.

Preface

This is a one-size-fits-all world. The current approach to nutrition is focused on cure-all panaceas that claim to be good for everyone. From the newest fad-diet craze to the latest super pill, pop culture has found its way into the world of nutrition. My life's work has focused on developing a natural, nutritional system of healing that safely, and effectively, addresses the needs of each and every person.

Customized Healing is a book that reflects this system I've developed over the past three decades. One of its components is my individualized healing method, electromagnetic muscle testing (EMT). It was inspired by the ancient Chinese five constitutional types theory and consists of a muscle-testing protocol that enables people to develop and maintain a pinpointed, customized nutrition plan. My EMT approach to customized healing has allowed many thousands to attain a greater level of health and balance, and overcome chronic illness and disease.

Customized Healing uses the Chinese system of the five constitutional types to personalize the basic dietary guidelines, thereby customizing food plans for individuals. To find out your particular type and the corresponding foods that are particularly good for you, refer to the questionnaire in Chapter 6 and to Chapters 5–12 on the individual types: wood, fire, earth, metal, and water. The book goes on to explain in greater detail how to arrive at your own personalized system of natural healing, and the back of the book includes a question-and-answer Appendix, a list of helpful Resources, relevant References, and an Index.

Customized Healing is a reflection of my life's work inspired by a truly remarkable, timeless, ancient system.

Acknowledgments

I would like to acknowledge:

Norman Goldfind, who had the vision to publish *Customized Healing;*

Nancy Dunn and Connie Mac Sweeney for their recipes;

Joel Price for his technical support;

Master Thomas Tam for his ta'i ch'i exercises;

Master Hua-Ching Ni for sharing his great wisdom;

Bobby Waddell for her superb editing assistance.

PART 1

Healing Depends On Wholeness

1

Redefining Health and Healing

Beyond the world of physical there is a higher,
spiritual realm of forms or ideas beyond matter or mechanism.

—PLATO

THE SPIRIT OF HEALING

For almost thirty years as a nutritional and holistic therapist, I have worked with tens of thousands of people. With every consultation, I have become increasingly aware that nature has equipped each of us with the ability to heal. It has also become clear that somewhere in the extreme of today's life, people have lost this ability.

But just exactly what is healing and why does it seem to be so elusive? I believe it is because of the quality of our lives. Take a break from your everyday attitudes for a moment to look deeply within, and there, beneath the surface of life, you'll find a force that animates, elevates, and fills everyone with energy. Although people are not often conscious of this inner aspect of being, it is unconsciously acknowledged when a particular person is noted as being "full of life," having "a lot of spirit," or "a good vibe." These comments all indicate a recognition of a transcendent, spiritlike quality in other human beings.

It is this spiritual essence that I believe holds the key to healing potential.

Although many talk about spirit, the truth is that, as a culture, most people have lost touch with it, along with their wholeness and an awareness of themselves as spiritual, not just physical, beings. In order to heal, it is first important to become whole. Yet without a spiritual sense of self—a sense of spirit and energy—people are left less than whole, disassociated, and out of touch with an integral part of themselves.

It's easy to see why this has happened. This culture's extremely materialistic bias maintains that only physical things are real, and it invalidates internal realities based on intuition, energy, feelings, and beliefs. Because of this, people have incorrectly defined spirituality and have often respond to it with misunderstanding and mistrust. A good many believe that spirituality is some amorphous thing that can only be found in religious institutions, or is something mystical and mysterious.

But spirituality is simpler than all that; it is as much a part of daily life as the air you breathe. Spirituality is all around everyone every day.

It's every aspect of the universe and of nature.

It is the inspiration that comes with the birth of a child, the joy that is felt with the coming of spring, or the grief felt at the death of a loved one.

Spirituality is reflected in the unique energy of each and every living thing.

Spirit is *everything* that is not material: life-force energy, dreams, hopes, beliefs, emotions.

Intuition, too, is a type of internal, spiritual phenomenon that science can't measure (maybe one day they'll figure out how—science can now measure many things it couldn't a century ago) and contemporary culture doesn't value. Consequently, unlike their ancestors, people don't trust themselves, their instincts, or what they know in their hearts to be true. This results in a division between the mind and the heart, the mind and the spirit. People may even say they care about soulful and spiritual phenomena, but often the bottom line is that they don't believe that things they *can't* see can affect them. People forget that they believe in plenty of energies that can't be seen: the forces that bring electricity into the home, the voices at the other end of the phone, the pictures and sound in TVs, computers, and the Internet.

This separation between hearts and minds—the denial of instinctive, intuitive, spiritual natures—creates a terrible rift in the fabric of human beings that has resulted in a grievous lack of self-integration and self-esteem. But how can anyone possibly find the key to trusting and loving themselves if they are disconnected from their true nature?

Herbert Maslow, the esteemed human behaviorist, taught that the greatest of all human needs is self-esteem. Greater than the need for food, shelter, or clothing is the need to establish a *true self-identity*. Without this, it is not possible determine values, priorities, or reasons for living. To love, to be whole, and to heal, every single person must know and be *who they are*.

The truth is that who people are is *not* just their material bodies, but also their souls, spirits, and minds.

Not everything can be measured by science yet, and not everything can be known, understood, or treated from the outside. Human beings are a miraculous complex of physical (material) and non-physical (spiritual) energy systems. Like the electricity that illuminates a light bulb, they are powered by an unseen energy life force.

To customize and maximize true healing potential, you need to begin by acknowledging this energy force as it expresses itself in the energies of your mind, spirit, and soul. These parts of yourself—your beliefs, intuitions, thoughts, feelings—must be cared for with as much attention as you devote to your physical body. You need to acknowledge that the body, mind, spirit, and soul are connected *in a practical sense*. You cannot hate or resent this connection and pretend that those feelings have nothing to do with your hypertension and indigestion. Every scientist and physician now realizes that those feelings have everything to do with physical health. No point keeping a stiff upper lip when your heart is heavy but is refusing to express the grief. Eventually, the grief will find physical expression because emotions are real and have the power to affect the workings of the body.

In physics, it's the relationship between energy and matter.

For the purposes of this book, I use the word *mind* to refer to the whole spectrum of this part of life-force energy—the spiritual phenomena that include emotions, intuition, thoughts, beliefs, and feelings.

As you become more tuned-in to these internal dynamics, you will come to more clearly distinguish between them. Begin by acknowledging their presence, their power, and the mysterious and wondrous aspect of life they represent. Without this acknowledgment, you can never be whole and you cannot heal.

THE SPIRIT OF *WHOLISM*

Just as people need to claim wholeness and the natural, right relationship with themselves as physical, mental, and spiritual beings, they also need to claim their rightful place in the world as a unique part of a greater whole. This awareness is all but lost in modern technological life.

Once, the ancient ancestors lived in tune with Nature. They knew who they were because they recognized their intimate relationships to the big, consistent cycles that brought seed in spring, growth in summer, bounty in fall. Westerners today, however, live as though they can conquer and dominate Nature with no detrimental effects. Technological prowess has led most people to believe they are in no way dependent upon, or connected to, the great cycles of birth and growth by which their ancestors lived and died. But everyone is a part of Nature, and Nature lives within everyone. It is not possible to prosper and remain separate from the natural world, for to do so is to remain severed from your own true natures.

To claim the power to heal, it is first necessary to reclaim awareness of *whole-ism*. As these fundamental changes in awareness filter down into your life, you begin to change the way you think. As you become whole, you will begin to question many of your previous assumptions.

Another result of living in a materialistic, externally focused culture is losing the belief that you can affect your own healing and thinking instead that only an external agent, a doctor in most cases, can fix you when you're sick. Yet, study after study, as well as the many personal histories being published today, show that people who take an active role in their own healthcare—prevention and treatment—have far more positive results than those who don't. Again, the problem involves changing the beliefs that denigrate the power of your energy by denigrating your own experiences, feelings, and intuitions.

This disinclination to trust your own healing instincts has been fostered by a mechanically biased culture and its medical philosophy that generally, and hypocritically, denies that any kind of life-force energy can have an effect on your health, even when that same medical establishment has plenty of studies to prove otherwise and has, in limited ways, acknowledged the relationship between such energy and health (stress leading to elevated blood pressure, heart attacks, or ulcers, for example).

And while some may believe that emotions wield some power in everyday life, it's likely still not understood how they can influence healing. To most, an inflammation remains an inflammation, and a cyst is just a cyst.

Just as it's important to acknowledge the need to be a good steward of your physical life force, you cannot ignore the effect of your emotional life on your health. You can't expect to be healthy in body, mind, and spirit if you don't pay attention to each of these. You need to give your body good fuel and regular exercise; mental health is maintained by exercising (in other words, acknowledging and releasing) your emotions, and by stimulating your mind; your spirit is nurtured with music, meditation, or spiritual practice. However you choose to live your life, you need to remind yourself often that these three elements—body, mind, and spirit—are *inseparable* elements of the *whole* human being.

FACING FEARS HELPS ED BEAT BACK ILLNESS

In my work as a nutitionist and practitioner of classic Chinese medicine, Ed, a patient in his sixties, came to see me after being diagnosed with a rare form of cancer. His doctors had told him he had three months to live. At the time of his diagnosis, Ed's daughter was due to graduate from UCLA in four month's time and he dearly wanted to be present. This presented him with a real problem because flying topped of the list of many immobilizing fears he had experienced throughout his life. But a few weeks later, the cancer diagnosis and his feeling that he no longer had anything to lose led him to decide he was not only *going* to live long enough to congratulate his daughter on her graduation, but he was going to get on an airplane for the first time in his life and *fly* to California from the East Coast to watch her graduate. Ed bought a round-trip ticket, and, challenging his most crippling fear, he flew to Los Angeles for her graduation. Shortly after his return—about five months after the doctors had given him his three-month death sentence—Ed's doctors found that his cancer had gone into full remission. Now, about a decade later, he remains healthy and cancer-free.

Everything you do (how you deal with stress, what you think, feel, and believe, how you choose and prepare the food you eat, the kinds of medicines you take, if any) creates an energetic response that either *enhances* or *diminishes* your life-force energy. You need to recognize that all parts of yourself—whether flesh, feeling, or faith—are different conduits for the same single animating life force.

VITALISTIC AND MECHANISTIC BELIEF SYSTEMS

What humankind knows and believes about healing and wellness has continually changed from the beginning of time. Healing systems also differ vastly from one culture to another. Although, except for Native Americans and native peoples in North, Central, and South America, people in the West have been steeped in today's material worldview, there is luckily another model to inform them. To learn from this model, you can look both to your own past and to the ancient healing system (still in use and well-studied and validated) of Eastern cultures, most notably India's ayurveda and classic Chinese medicine (CCM), which has been my dominant influence.

This model is based on the premise that all life is endowed with a vitalizing life force, an energy that both animates matter *and* forms it. In this model, human beings are part of the natural world and subject to its laws.

Vitalism, as this system is called, holds that although man participates in the process, *it is Nature that ultimately heals.* Health, then, is matter of complying with Nature in order to most beneficially cultivate the life force that flows through everyone.

Perhaps you can remember your grandparents, or the woman up the street, or the old family doctor as vitalists. When you were sick, they would have wanted to know what was going on at school, how you were feeling, whether you'd gotten a chill at recess. They might have asked what you'd eaten for breakfast, whether you'd been properly dressed for the weather, what was happening at home recently and before you left for school. They innately understood that human beings were whole mind/body systems comprised of interwoven energies that profoundly affected health. They ministered to your feelings and asked about your interaction with your world. They knew that good health was affected by, and the result of, adapting to the dictates of Nature—both inside and out.

On the other hand, the materialistic philosophy of today can be described as a mechanistic system. *Mechanism* is distinguished by its belief that people are separate from nature: the human mind and spirit can be separated from the body and, like machines, can be analyzed and treated in isolation from nature.

Although mechanistic philosophy (which formed the basis of the Western scientific medical model) still dominates thinking, contemporary science continues to move beyond it. The advanced study of physics has established that all of life can be reduced to a common element billions of times smaller than an atom. Quanta, as they are called by physicists, are neither matter nor energy, but a kind of basic essence from which both are formed. When reduced to its smallest parts, then, the entire phenomenal world is comprised of the same basic stuff.

The science of subatomic physics has established that humans are *not* separate from each other or from Nature, but are *connected* in one vast energetic field. This is quantum field theory, and it is a first cousin to vitalism.

Science, then, has proven what the ancients (and even the more *recents*) intuitively knew to be true. This mechanistic-style validation of vitalistic principles is a greater validation of whole-ism.

Reclaiming Intuitive Knowledge

In the past twenty-five years or so, bolstered by the success of science in *proving* what had always been essentially intuitive knowledge, the Western world has begun to reclaim a more vitalistic model of living and healing. Many techniques from vitalistic medicinal systems have begun to filter into the everyday world, and alternative therapies and complementary medicine are becoming more and more common. Today, there are many programs at respected medical centers that use a variety of preventive techniques to treat illnesses. Nutritional therapy, as well as mind/body medicine (which includes such stress-reduction techniques as breathing, meditation, ta'i ch'i, and yoga exercises) have proven themselves effective in treating a vast array of medical problems. A host of double-blind studies—the only way Westerners will really believe something is true—illustrate how cultivation and manipulation of the life-force energy heals disease and creates vibrant health.

Not long ago, a study of Finnish men indicated that those who didn't feel love or hope were 20 percent more likely to die of cancer than those men who did. Equally fascinating is the research being done at the Institute of Heartmath, a think tank in Santa Cruz, California. Researchers there are monitoring changes in the bodies of subjects as they practice simple exercises that focus loving feelings in the heart. Not only does the actual heartbeat change in a matter of minutes, but these changes dramatically raise the body's levels of anti-aging hormones, strengthen several chemical indicators of immune-system function, balance the sympathetic and parasympathetic nervous systems, and lower a hormone that promotes aging and illness.

Every day, the evidence is mounting to prove that a life-force energy profoundly affects the course of the physical body. What the ancient Chinese knew 5,000 years ago is now better understood—that health and illness are not random events, but are largely the result of how naturally the life-force energy is cultivated.

Of course, knowledge is one thing; incorporating it into your life is another. Experience brings belief, and belief calls for more experience. In order to begin to harness your true healing power, you need to alter how you view who you are and what you believe. Perhaps looking at the world through the eyes of a higher consciousness can be your greatest healing experience.

FIXING KATHY'S DEBILITATING FOOD SENSITIVITIES

One of my patient's stories is particularly vivid in my mind. At the time I worked with Kathy, she was a young woman in her early thirties who had experienced extreme food sensitivities for several years. There were very few foods she could tolerate without getting sick. She became so congested when she ate dairy, wheat, and yeast that she couldn't function. She also had a number of immunological problems. I muscle-tested her (*see* Chapter 14) and weaned her from the foods to which she showed sensitivity. Kathy came to the office frequently—once a week for the first month, then every two or three weeks.

During the four months I worked with Kathy, we got to know each other better. Eventually she told me that she'd been living with her fiancé for ten years and wanted to get married, but he didn't. She never mentioned it to him though, for fear of losing him. As time passed, she began to feel increasingly bothered by the fact that she wasn't telling him how she felt. We talked about this, and I gently urged her to stand up for herself, her needs, and her feelings. I stressed that I thought it was important for her to express herself. Eventually, she mustered up the conviction and confronted him. Although he remained unmoved by this honest expression of her needs, she stood her ground and a short while later they split up. Kathy was initially upset by this turn of events, but almost immediately all her food sensitivities disappeared. When we met in the weeks following the breakup, she was sad, but felt free from the fear that had bound her for years. She had liberated her heart, and her heart had liberated her body of its debilitating symptoms.

Kathy's story underlines how everyone's life-force energy resides in their hearts, their cells, and their thoughts and beliefs. Whether your heart hurts from sadness and grief, or from blocked arteries, it is still *all* blocked energy. Natural healing involves cultivating and enhancing all your life-force energy, whether it's through the foods you eat, the kinds of medicines you use, what you think, how you act, or what you believe.

PUTTING IT ALL TOGETHER/THE MIND-BODY

In energetic terms then, there is no difference between the mind and the body. When a client comes to me with an ailment, it is necessary to look at all the influences that affect the problem. This means I look at the entire mind/body environment, since in a whole system, everything is related to everything. Only by blending the best of Western, mechanistic, and chemical knowledge with the best of the ancient and current vitalistic approach can you become a whole being and claim your maximum healing potential.

2

The Power to Heal

From wonder into wonder,
existence opens.

—LAO TZU

Concurrent with my thirty years of formal education, research, and practice in the science of nutrition, I have been a student of the art of Chinese medicine. Although nutritional therapy represents the primary focus of my life's work, my understanding and practice of Chinese medicine has dramatically changed the way I work. Nourishing the body with the proper foods isn't the only way to good health. Nourishing the mind is equally important.

In most cases, regardless of a client's illness, disharmonies need to be addressed on the mental-emotional level before they can be addressed on the physical. In order for healing to take place, the patient must *first* be viewed as whole.

Along with India's ayurveda, Chinese medicine was one of the first formalized medical systems to establish healing protocols that were mind/body oriented. Inspired and influenced by the Chinese approach to healing, my work isn't limited to one-dimensional nutritional therapy—it's an integrative, holistic approach.

CLASSICAL CHINESE MEDICINE VS. TRADITIONAL CHINESE MEDICINE—A VITAL DISTINCTION

It is important to point out that there are two distinctly different kinds of Chinese medicine. In all my books and in all the work I do, I only use *classical* Chinese medicine. Traditional Chinese medicine (TCM) is an outgrowth of classical Chinese medicine (CCM) that has been adapted for the mechanistic Western world.

Both the technological West and whatever Communist East remains share a mechanistic proclivity that ignores the mystical and spiritual roots so integral to CCM—I suspect that the potentially empowering mystical and spiritual aspects of CCM have frightened away the mechanists of the world. CCM teaches that there is a limitless flow of life-force power that resides with the tao (the source) and it is eternally available to anyone dedicated to a life of integral cultivation, a label that refers to proper diet and daily exercise, as well as a spiritual and mystical understanding.

TCM, on the other hand, merely inserts aspects of Chinese medicine into the branches of Western medicine, and therefore focuses on the mechanical. By contrast, in CCM the spirit is core.

Recently, there has been renewed interest in restoring classical Chinese medicine to its rightful place. There is a growing movement both in the East and here in the West that seeks to reinstate CCM as the more time-honored, authentic form of Chinese medicine. There are those who understand that without the mystical and the spiritual, there is simply no connection to the vital source that is the origin of all life force. Classical Chinese medicine takes into account the entirety of its history. The classical approach compares the old with the new styles and searches for the roots in the same tradition of the original founders.

Another key point is evolution. Ancient CCM wasn't standardized or regulated by any medical boards, and it wasn't the same from one year to the next, nor from one province to another. CCM always was, and forever remains, in a state of constant flow. It is ever-evolving from one practitioner and one family system to another. It changes and grows as its students change and grow. A remarkable discovery on any one given day in any one practitioner's life is merely added to the collective-consciousness archive, forever to be shared only within that specific practitioner's experience and cycled through the resonance of what Rupert Sheldrak called "morphic fields."

The healing system I developed and continue to practice employs classical Chinese medicine in real time, from moment to moment, one experience at a time. This allows the practitioner and the patient to observe and follow the stream of higher consciousness, allowing it to guide an awareness of those roots and origins of imbalance that keep them from wholeness and wellness. Classical Chinese medicine has always been up close, personal, and very much alive, and it always will be.

Any system that espouses wholism, yet omits taking the mystical and spiritual equally into account with the physical and mechanical, is simply *not* whole. People are complex, multifaceted beings with an endless variety of needs. In order to truly address the full scope of these healing needs, systems of medicine must open up to the limitless possibilities for the ever-changing intricacies of each and every patient. Every one of us remains a separate, complex, dynamic universe living within an ever-changing field of possibilities. Classical Chinese medicine clearly understood this, as it evolved from it. As is usually the case, history has a great deal to teach, in this case not only about who we were, but about who we truly *are* and always *will* be.

It is important to note here that ancient classical Chinese medicine has never been extremely standardized. Rather, it is an artful science that has been customized by each person who practices it. The knowledge has been passed down through the generations from family to family, each altering and adding to it. My understanding and application of Chinese medicinal principles is very much in keeping with this. I have developed a hybrid of ancient classical Chinese healing arts and current techniques in all of the therapies I use. In my dietary work, for instance, I blend the latest in nutritional, chemical knowledge with the classical Chinese approach, a customized system based on the energetic properties of food, something I will discuss in more detail later in the book.

Classical Chinese medicine encompasses eight healing arts, known today as the *Eight Strands of the Brocade.* These eight, which have been passed from family to family over the centuries, make up the primary pillars of Chinese medicine. Each one is a model of energy healing: nutrition, herbal therapy (natural medicines), occlusion (mind/body medicine), contact thermogenesis (energy healing), acupressure, acupuncture, diagnosis, and massage.

I work with four of the eight, and this book will focus on the following three: nutritional therapy, mind/body medicine, and natural medicine, which today includes vitamins and minerals.

Before delving into these basic therapeutic approaches, I will take a closer look at the fundamental belief systems of classical Chinese medicine (CCM).

SIMPLIFIED FUNDAMENTALS
OF CLASSICAL CHINESE MEDICINE

The ancient Chinese belief system begins with the idea that all of life exists within the web of Nature. In this context, all things are interconnected and interdependent. Events influence all parts within a whole concurrently: what is good for one part is good for all because everything and everyone is part of the same whole.

This way of thinking is reflected in the ancient Chinese approach to health and healing, which sees symptoms in relationship to the whole mind/body and sees human beings in relationship to all of Nature. Therefore, good health is the result of healthy interactions among all parts and systems of the mind-body.

Allopathic (Western) medicine, on the other hand, targets specific sets of symptoms and treats them with synthetic pharmaceuticals and other treatments, including surgery, as though they exist in isolation from the rest of the mind/body.

Often, however, Western medications have unhealthy, even life-threatening side effects. They can have an impact on bodily processes and functions other than the one(s) they are targeting, ignoring the fact that symptoms cannot be treated as though one part of the mind/body doesn't affect another. Additionally, instead of treating the cause, Western medicines frequently treat or mask symptoms, thereby producing a false sense of wellness. When this happens, rather than addressing the cause and making lifestyle or dietary changes, the person does nothing and thinks he or she is cured. In this case, the problem that the illness reflected can take hold of the person on an even deeper level because the needs of the mind/body haven't been addressed or fulfilled, just masked. From the Chinese point of view, symptoms are seen as messages that communicate important information about what the mind/body needs.

SARAH'S STORY—IN HER OWN WORDS

I had been living with a diagnosis of MS (multiple sclerosis) for about six years. After years of playing around with Western medicine, I didn't know what to do. I'd never been sick before in my life and I was stuck with multiple sclerosis. Thank God I'm a die-hard optimist because it was such a dead end. Every three months I'd end up in the hospital for 10 days of steroids. Then I'd get sent home and I'd feel sicker than when I went in. It was the side effects. After a while, I realized that the side effects of the drugs were killing me.

At one point, someone said to me, 'Why don't you look into holistic medicine?' So I asked around and I kept hearing the name Mark Mincolla. One day, after I'd left a message at his office, but hadn't heard back from him yet, I was in the natural food store and who should come in but Mark Mincolla and his wife. So I started going to him.

Mark took my history. He's holistic, so he had to know the whole story—when I got sick, how I got sick, what was going on in my life. I was very stressed at work, and I was a very career-minded person.

Every month, I went to see Mark. Right away, he changed my diet. He felt he could put out the fire in my legs, and he did. Then I started getting bladder infections, and the doctors put me on antibiotics. I couldn't break that cycle of antibiotic dependency, until finally, with Mark's diet and therapies, the antibiotic-induced infections finally went away.

I continue to follow the diet he put me on—low-fat, mostly vegetables and proteins. He also has me on supplements. Sometimes I cheat with food a little bit—I take the 10 percent leeway he allows me—but I'm feeling better, to the point where I recently went back to work. I was overwhelmed with enthusiasm to be working again. Mark has helped me follow a different route to a long-lasting career. Now, I firmly let my limits be known and speak my mind when something is bothering me. I've learned how to say *no* when it's appropriate and I work at my own pace, based on what I'm feeling and not on what I think everyone else expects of me.

It is great to be able to play the game of life once again and not have to watch from the sidelines. I am happy Mark is the manager of my team. He helped me understand that I needed to change the rules a bit to make the game both enjoyable and winnable. It's a small miracle, really.

Throughout the course of our work together, Sarah clearly learned that all the events of her life had profoundly influenced her mind and her body. I have never seen anyone work harder at respecting and positively reprogramming her subtle mind/body energies. She continues to prosper in good health.

Ch'i

Perhaps the most fundamental concept of classical Chinese medicine is the idea that all nature is powered by ch'i, a life-force energy.

All events and things are powered by ch'i and are made of ch'i. It represents form *and* process, matter *and* energy. Ch'i is the wind that blows and the trees that bend. It is the rising of the sap and the forming of chlorophyll. Ch'i is the instinct that sends the salmon upstream to lay its eggs. It is apparent in gravity, magnetism, and electricity. Ch'i is the life energy that *moves* everyone and the flesh that *is* everyone.

- The first law of Chinese medicine states that ch'i is ever-present and everywhere.

- The second law of Chinese Medicine states that ch'i is in constant motion. Never stopping, it is the nature of ch'i to continuously cycle between polar and complementary opposites: cold and hot, winter and summer, beginning and end, yin and yang. This constant movement represents *all* potential energy patterns, movements, and expressions in nature. When ch'i is balanced and centered, life is in harmony. Since the natural state of ch'i is movement, it follows that something is wrong when movement becomes blocked. You can see countless examples of this in both the mind and the body—whether cholesterol blocks circulation or repression blocks the flow of a particular emotion, both result in disease.

• The third law of Chinese medicine states exactly this—when ch'i is blocked, there is disharmony. Translated into a healing context, this means that when ch'i, or energy, is out of balance or blocked, disease results.

DISEASE AS MESSENGER

Just as health is the natural result of a balanced condition in the body, illness is the natural result of an imbalance.

Illnesses are messengers indicating that the mind/body needs something. If you ignore what these messengers are communicating, increasingly serious illnesses will result. From Chinese medicine you learn that imbalances or problems travel from one organ system to another if they are left uncorrected. What begins as an easily treated, simple illness can become a serious illness. Mildly troubling symptoms can turn into chronic and acute illness if the original problem is left untreated.

Western medicine would have you believe that you either have a disease or you don't. Most often, though, diseases develop over time when unfavorable conditions remain untreated. Chronic energy swings after too much sugar, for example, will inevitably develop into disease as time passes. I have often heard people blame the medical establishment for not correctly diagnosing them with a chronic condition, but these people don't understand that they had not yet developed the full range of symptoms recognizable as the particular disease. Most often, the person has ignored how they've felt for years and has

failed to make dietary, lifestyle, or other changes that would have alle-
viated their symptoms and reversed their progression toward a disease. Having failed to heed these messages, they eventually do develop
a serious illness.

The mind/body first attempts to communicate in symptomatic whis-
pers. If you fail to listen, however, it will scream and shout. Self-care and
learning to listen to your body is fundamental to maximizing your health
and healing potential. You must learn to recognize and respond to the
body's subtlest communications.

HEALING IS A NATURAL STATE

It is natural for ch'i to be life-giving, just as it is natural that bodies heal.
The minute you cut yourself, the wound begins to heal. Thousands of
processes immediately mobilize to start their healing work.

All of Nature is endowed with this self-regulating spirit of renewal.
Even the Earth as a whole is seen as a single entity with these abilities.
The *Gaia Hypothesis,* set forth by the British scientist James Lovelock
postulates that the Earth is a living being that can mobilize a multitude
of processes to counteract the changing influences to which it is continually subject. This allows the planet to maintain its equilibrium, despite
the natural changes to which she must continually adapt. And this
reflects the fundamental Chinese philosophy that an organism's ability
to adapt to changing conditions is the single most important measure
of its good health.

In the crush of technology and the external focus that has characterized recent culture, most Westerners have lost a sense of being connected
to Nature. They are part of the Earth, though, and the same forces that
operate in Nature operate in them. Each person is a microcosm, a smaller
version, of the Earth as a whole. They are part of the Earth, just as the
Earth is part of the universe. These patterns in Nature reveal the underlying connection with the universe. Existence is revealed as a set of carved
Chinese boxes, each one nestled inside the next: there are stars, comets,
and planets within the universe; humanity, seas, and fire within the Earth;
blood, mind, and spirit within humanity; and electrons, protons, and

nuclei within atoms. The world is comprised of a vast and never-ending whole of interconnected parts that each have corresponding cycles, processes, and tendencies. And just as the sailor learns to navigate the currents of wind and water to his best advantage, you must recognize yourself as part of the natural world and learn to adapt to its dictates.

Natural law is innately understood on the most basic level. For instance, if you eat nothing, you will eventually die; if you eat too much, you will gain weight. If you try to stay awake, you will eventually fall asleep; if you try too hard to sleep, you will stay awake.

There are many other laws, and Chinese medicine contains a wealth of wisdom about them. Their medicine is the result of thousands of years of observing Nature and detailing its way. To know the ways of Nature is to know how to balance, cultivate, and consequently enhance your life-force energy—ch'i.

The Chinese have classified many characteristics of ch'i. The following section contains a very brief overview that will spark your innate understanding of the energy that continuously flows through you.

YIN AND YANG AND THE FIVE ENERGIES

All of Nature arises from a single unified oneness. From this oneness, referred to as the *tao* (God The Way), comes all being that is differentiated from the oneness by the very fact that it has a separate identity. Beingness—everything that can be spoken of and named—is made up of opposites: night and day, tall and short, full and empty, internal and external, cold and hot. These complementary poles both form and define all things. It is impossible to know light without darkness, front without back, hot without cold, sorrow without joy.

These archetypal extremes are referred to as yin and yang.

Although yin and yang are opposites, they are complementary parts of a single whole and they balance each other. These complementary opposites are constantly interweaving, as day gives way to night, up to down, movement to stillness. One aspect is continually changing into another. Yin is constantly changing into yang, and yang is constantly changing into yin. After the pendulum swings to its most extreme point, it moves in the other direction, as exemplified by the saying that the darkest hour is just before dawn.

The Chinese use yin and yang to describe the cyclical nature of the world through complementary opposites, and they further divide the world into *Five Energies:* Just as the seasons flow from one to the other, *Wood, Fire, Earth, Metal,* and *Water* are used to organize and understand the underlying energy movement and cyclical development of all things, from beginning to end and back again. The five energies have a variety of corresponding aspects to them that can be applied to people, places, foods, herbs, processes, and ideas.

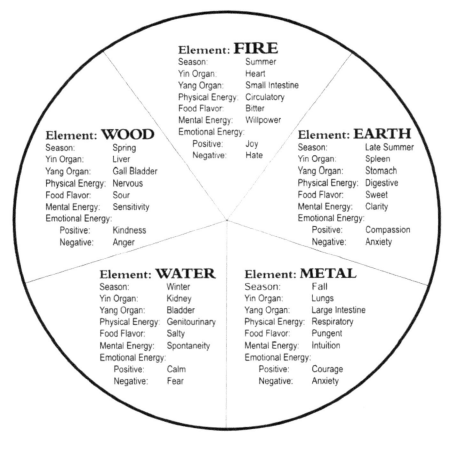

Properties of the Five Energies.

THE FIVE ENERGIES

I use the Five Energies as a tool for customizing nutritional therapy by matching the five constitutional types with the corresponding food flavors that maximize their healing potential. (*See* Chapter 14.)

The Ways of Energy—How Power Moves

Just as the Earth experiences the forces of Nature, so, too, do human beings. Ch'i, which encompasses these forces, is in constant movement, cycling from one pole to the other in a continuous ebb and flow. By understanding the nature of ch'i, you can help facilitate its unfettered movement. In keeping with this, the Chinese classified many forms, characteristics, attributes, and movements of ch'i in order to manipulate and balance their vital life force.

THE FOUR SOURCES OF CH'I

Ch'i is derived from four sources:

1. The process of respiration receives ch'i from oxygen.

2. The process of digestion receives ch'i from food.

3. The process of circulation receives ch'i from the blood.

4. The process of excretion receives ch'i from detoxification.

These sources help Westerners better understand the practical aspects of ch'i. Oxygen, for instance, is understood by both East and West as the most vital source of all life-giving power. It is easy to grasp the role it plays in health and healing. Science says that as much as 75 percent of the human body is comprised of water, and 90 percent of water is comprised of oxygen.

When the body receives the correct amount of oxygen, it is able to create carbon dioxide in the proper ratios, forming a gas the body can eliminate. This process of oxidation allows the body to maintain a normal temperature that fortifies the immune capabilities of the glands and organs. On the other hand, if oxygen is not sufficiently supplied to the bloodstream, carbon monoxide is formed and is not readily eliminated from the body, thus upsetting the maintenance of normal body temperatures. This situation allows a multitude of environmental stresses to invade the glands and organs, setting the stage for disease.

Just like oxygen, food (through digestion) is also a primary carrier of ch'i. Although Western medicine is in the early stages of working with nutrition medicinally, the ancient Chinese classified it as one of their healing modalities as well as one of the primary sources of ch'i.

THE SIX MANIFESTATIONS OF CH'I

When ch'i moves, it manifests in some form or another. There are six manifestations of naturally directed ch'i:

1. When ch'i congeals, it creates matter.

2. When ch'i disperses, it creates space.

3. When ch'i animates, it creates life.

4. When ch'i flows, it creates health.

5. When ch'i is blocked, it creates sickness.

6. When ch'i departs, it creates death.

(*My understanding of the Four Sources and The Six Manifestations of Ch'i were taught to me by Master Hua-Ching Ni.*)[1]

In the true spirit of Chinese medicine, the primary focus of my work is to enhance the flowing manifestation of ch'i while avoiding the blockage of ch'i.

When ch'i flows there is health; when ch'i is blocked, there is disease.

For example, cholesterol blockages can, in most cases, be treated successfully with diet and/or natural medicines because reducing the intake of saturated fat rids the arteries of plaque deposits and allows the blood to flow freely. Fish oils, lecithin, and niacin (vitamin B_3) aid in this process. In some cases, natural medicines, such as these, along with dietary modifications, are all that is necessary to reverse the condition.

To relieve ailments, problems need to be addressed on the physical, emotional, and energy levels. In many cases, it isn't only physical reasons that prevent an organ or bodily system from maintaining a balanced wellness. Often, there are unresolved emotional issues that further block the flow of ch'i to the point of dysfunction.

The five emotions system is very instructive in this. Emotional energy is a real force that must be released and expressed. If it isn't released externally, it will be stored in the body. (*See* Chapters 7–11 for specific correspondences between emotions and organ systems.)

Just as the heart becomes diseased from a blockage of ch'i-giving blood, the lungs become diseased if they are blocked from receiving oxygen through a breakdown in the process of respiration. Asthma is an ailment commonly linked in the West to both emotional and physical blockages. This parallels the Chinese belief that unexpressed grief stores in the lungs if not properly expressed. In this case, mind/body protocols must be employed to ensure recovery. And diet is frequently a contributing factor. I've had hundreds of patients whose asthma has been relieved when dairy is restricted or eliminated. Dairy products create phlegm and mucus that often blocks the lungs, obstructing respiration. Again, you have to look at the whole person to see which factors are at work.

The goal is to find ways to facilitate the movement of ch'i, or energy, within the body. Nutrition is a wonderful tool for this.

Using digestion and assimilation as examples, many people are unable to break down calcium because of inadequate hydrochloric (digestive) acids in the stomach. When the body cannot break calcium down, it must be stored someplace, frequently as kidney stones or arterial blockages, so this is a serious (and common) problem.

Interestingly, stress is often the first culprit in the inability to break calcium down. When the body is stressed, the adrenal glands chemically stress the thyroid gland, causing it to stop producing calcitonin, calcium's digestive hormone. This cycle can initiate an array of problems, since digestion is vital for unlocking nutrients from the foods that contain them.

Often, you can work backward from symptoms to find where the body's natural processes were blocked from doing their job. In many cases, Western allopathic medicines mask the real problem, causing the body to become more and more out of balance, setting the stage for more complex levels of dysfunction.

In the next chapter, I will give a brief overview of the three healing brocades (taoist exercises) that make up the customized healing of the book's title. They are:

1. Nutritional therapy;

2. Natural medicines; and

3. Mind/body medicine.

I believe these three approaches can be used as the core conduits of ch'i to maximize your healing potential.

The New Medicine—
Blending East and West
for Customized Healing

In many ways, Western medicine and ancient classical Chinese medicine are opposites. Yet you can see how well they work together. Their mutual compatibility exemplifies the well-known concept of yin and yang. On the simplest level, yin and yang are symbols for any two polar opposites that comprise a single whole, and Eastern and Western medicine represent two sides of the same coin.

As culture becomes more global, the view of the world changes. Where once people only identified with the those closest to them, they now identify with the wider world as a part of themselves. In the same way, Eastern and Western medicines, previously worlds apart, are beginning to come together. Now, stress management and other mind/body approaches to healing are as critical to heart health as any cholesterol medication. Although the Western allopathic medical model still has a very strong foothold, things are changing, and a new hybrid—complementary medicine—is emerging that blends the best of the Eastern and Western systems.

PREVENTION

Eastern and Western models combine to create a much more complete healing system than either one alone. The most important contribution Eastern medicine has made to the Western way of thinking is its focus on prevention.

Prevention involves supporting and enhancing the body's own natural healing system as the first line of defense against disease. As sensible and simple as this approach is, only in the past twenty years has it attracted the attention of Western medicine, which is predominantly disease-oriented and applied only *after* illness has already occurred. But why not keep illness from happening in the first place?

The Western medical system is more about politics, economics, and corporate profit than it is about health. There is a lot more money to be made treating illness rather than preventing it, or even curing it.

Even so, there is a lot of truth in the old maxim that an ounce of prevention is worth a pound of cure. It really is much better and easier to make a consistent effort to be healthy than to fight disease.

Just as efficiency experts emulate the habits of successful entrepreneurs, medical researchers would do well to study the habits of healthy people and learn from them. So many research dollars have gone into devising ways to attack disease, while little effort is expended in learning how to prevent it. It's as if they've spent all their time studying the habits of the enemy rather than reinforcing the walls of the body's precious immune fortress. When you focus so much attention on healthcare being disease-oriented rather than wellness-oriented, it's hard to take prevention seriously. But all that is changing.

The Amazing Healing System

The goal of prevention is to fortify the body's natural ability to fend off disease before it has a chance to take hold. This approach has grown out of the awareness that healing is a natural function of the body. Not only does the body have an amazing immune system defending itself against ever-present viruses, cancers, and bacteria, but it is also engaged in an ongoing process of self-repair. From the unseen realms to the most obvious cuts and breaks, the body's intelligence is at work.

The immune system, comprised of trillions of specialized cells, has three main types of T-cells (immune cells). One group, the killer T-cells, constantly patrols the body searching out foreign invaders. When a killer T-cell encounters a virus, tumor, bacteria, or other micro-enemy, it communicates this information to another group of cells called helper T-cells, which have several strategies for destroying a foreign body: after these Pacman-like cells destroy the invader's walls, they surround the enemy with their spider-like tentacles and release enzymes that disman-tle the cell's component parts. These remarkable cells then study the dead invader and transmit chemical alarms throughout the body that teach other immune cells how to recognize and remember the invaders. These specialized memory cells then remember the invader's character-istics for the rest of the person's life. If the memory cells encounter the invader again, even years later, they are able to recognize it very quickly and can alert the killer T-cells immediately. After this cellular search-and-destroy mission is completed, another group called suppressor T-cells arrive to call off the fight and clean up the debris.

The body continually hosts a multitude of foreign invaders, includ-ing cancer cells, bacteria, viruses, fungi, and various allergens capable of creating disease. Only a healthy and vigorous immune system is able to resist their advance. This is where diet and natural medicines come in—they directly affect the production and potency of immune cells, the majority of which are white blood cells. This is why it is so important to nourish and enhance all the components of the immune system. And, since all bodily systems are connected to each other (like the old song about the hip bone being connected to the thigh bone), whatever is good for any one part or system of the body ultimately enhances the working of the entire immune system.

The thymus gland, which produces tens of millions of T-cells every minute, is one of the primary components of the immune system. Bone marrow, too, produces millions of white blood cells that act as primary immune cells, while the spleen, the lymph nodes, and the ducts produce a variety of proteins and chemical messengers, such as interferon, which kill invaders such as ever-present cancer cells. No matter what therapies, drugs, or surgery a person may use to cure a disease, when all is said and done, *it is the body's own healing system that does the work.*

When disease has taken a very strong hold, the body's healing and immune systems have been overwhelmed and disabled. Then invasive therapies work by destroying enough of the diseased parts to allow the healing system to cope with the rest and come back online. The tricky part of using invasive therapies is that they can, and frequently do, destroy the very cells, tissues, and organs of the immune system that are so critically important for healing.

Many studies today illustrate just how effectively nutritional support can protect the immune system while a body undergoes chemotherapy, radiation, or antibiotics. These drastic therapies are not smart bombs; they don't just target the cancer or infected cells, they go after healthy cells as well. Antibiotics, for instance, kill off a large population of the body's good bacteria along with the invasive ones. That's why it is important to eat acidophilus and other active bacterial cultures (found in yogurt) to restore the beneficial flora when taking antibiotics.

Studies indicate that, in cancer patients undergoing radiation treatments, vitamins C, E, and other antioxidants can protect vital immune organs while also enhancing tumor reduction. Vitamin E also protects the heart from damage caused by adriamycin, a chemotherapy drug, and it seems to have an anti-cancer component as well. These antioxidant nutrients are found abundantly in fresh fruits and vegetables, especially those with the darkest colors. (*See* Chapter 15 for detailed information on antioxidants in foods.) Many other studies, including those performed by Linus Pauling (his Nobel prize was awarded for his research on vitamin C), indicate that cancer patients who undergo nutritional support live longer and do better than those who do not.

There has been much recent controversy over the safety and effectiveness of vitamin E since the Hope Too Study was released, suggesting that vitamin E was of no real value regarding heart disease. This study implied that people who take the vitamin in supplement form may actually tend to die earlier. Annette Dickenson, Ph.D., the spokesperson for The Council for Responsible Nutrition, was quick to point out that the Hope Too study was very poorly constructed. She said the study was flawed because it selected unhealthy candidates over age seventy. Those who are unhealthy and older are often more inclined to take vitamin supplements out of desperation. To assume they died because of the vitamin supplement would be irresponsible. Once challenged, the study's authors agreed that their study's design could have been much better.

Professor Balz Frie of the Linus Pauling Institute at Oregon State University completed a study on free-radical biology and medicine in the fall of 2007 showing that generations of vitamin E studies may be meaningless. The study concluded that the levels of vitamin E necessary to reduce oxidative stress—as measured by accepted biomarkers of lipid peroxidation—are approximately 1,600–3,400 IU per day. That's four–eight times the doses studied to date. Frie, one of the world's leading experts on antioxidants and disease, stated there are a number of animal and human studies clearly demonstrating that vitamin E can inhibit atherosclerotic lesions, slow aortic thickening, lower inflammation, and reduce platelet adhesion via oxidative stress reduction.

The Linus Pauling Institute has a superb website where they document the history of viable studies demonstrating that vitamin C lowers the risks for cardiovascular disease, cataracts, certain cancers, diabetes, hypertension, and strokes, and counteracts the ill effects of both lead poisoning and the common cold.

IN ALICE'S OWN WORDS—PAIN WAS THE MAJOR MOTIVATOR FOR IMPROVING HER HEALTH

For two or three years before going to Mark, I'd been having severe abdominal pain. I couldn't sleep at night. I was trying to live with it . . . you put up with what you have to . . . until I started bleeding from the bowel and ended up in the hospital. When I left, my doctor told me I had to have an extensive operation, even though they weren't sure it would be successful. I didn't know what to do.

Meanwhile, my daughter had been going to Mark and had been trying to get me to go. Pain is a great motivator, so finally I went to see him. I was really in tough shape. Besides the bowel problem, I had very high blood pressure and I'd already had cancer, so I didn't need anything else. I didn't know how he was going to help me, but I went anyway.

Right away he changed my diet extensively. It seemed all the things I was told to use when I left the hospital were absolutely the opposite of what I could tolerate. I couldn't take regular bread or any milk products—I still can't take them, though I can have one type of bread:

sourdough rice bread. My basic diet now is low-fat proteins, like chicken, and various combinations of high-starch and low-starch vegetables. He put me on various supplements, and the pain left, finally. It took a little while, but it went away. It's gone.

So, I'm on a strict diet now and I follow it. It's been a year that my pain is gone and I feel so good. Can you believe it? I'm so grateful to him, I owe him my life. I was also on two blood pressure pills a day because my blood pressure was so high—I'd already had a stroke—but after I'd been going to Mark for about six months, my doctor lowered the dosage from two pills to one. My husband says my blood pressure is like a kid's now.

I see Mark about every six to eight weeks. Once, when I went to see my doctor, he was a little concerned because I'd lost weight, but of course I wasn't eating any sweets or anything since going to Mark. When I explained to the doctor that I was out of pain, he said, "Look, anything that works that well, just keep doing that." And that's what I do.

P.S. Alice no longer needs to see me on a regular basis, and she continues to thrive in good health.

It is even more effective, however, to support your precious immune system and enhance your life-force energy with good nutrition, natural medicine, and mind-body behavior techniques to prevent sickness. The following section gives an overview of these basic immune-enhancing approaches, which comprise the bulk of this book, beginning with a look at the Standard American Diet (SAD).

THE SAD (STANDARD AMERICAN DIET) TRUTH

Until very recently, the idea of food as medicine has been profoundly dismissed by our culture. Although the Academy of Sciences in the U.S. declared nutrition a science only in the 1960s, the Chinese have considered it a primary medicinal therapy for thousands of years.

In 1976, the United States Senate published a comprehensive study on nutrition, based on the testimony of 1,100 scientists from eight countries. The Select Committee on Nutrition and Human Needs, chaired by then Senator George McGovern, concluded that much of the sickness and disease in the U.S. was directly linked to diet. The most indicting testimony came from Dr. D. Mark Hegstead, head of the Harvard School of Public Health. Hegstead claimed that six of the leading ten causes of premature death in the U.S. are the direct result of the Standard American Diet, appropriately referred to as SAD.

In the three decades since this Senate Committee convened, a tremendous amount of research has confirmed and expanded its findings. Today, although the majority of Americans have yet to embrace the idea that diet is fundamental to health, a growing segment of the population is getting the message.

Perhaps a reality check is in order to realize how much diets have changed since the days when your parents or grandparents were kids. In the past century, the composition of the average diet in the U.S. has degenerated radically. The complex carbohydrates—fruits, vegetables, legumes, and grain products—that were the healthy mainstay of diets in your grandparents' time now, unfortunately, play a minor role. The fast food that now dominates the food culture didn't come on the scene until the '60s. Nor were there the massive number of convenience foods, packed with processed fats, sugars, and salt, that there are today. As a result, the consumption of saturated fats and sugar has risen to the point where these two dietary elements alone comprise at least 60 percent of the total caloric intake of Americans.

This amounts to a wave of malnutrition, from both over- and under-consumption.

The over-consumption of saturated fat and animal fat, in particular, is responsible for six of the leading ten causes of untimely death, among them heart disease, cancer, cerebrovascular disease, diabetes, and atherosclerosis.

The under-consumption of good sources of low-fat protein, essential fatty acids, and complex carbohydrates, including fruits, vegetables, and whole grains, deprives the body of the essential nutrients it needs.

This is particularly disturbing when you consider that today's children were born into the world of drive-through dining and processed convenience foods and have had this type of unhealthy diet from day one.

The American Academy of Pediatrics recently recommended that 200,000 American children between the ages of six and seventeen be put on cholesterol drugs. Their recommendation was the result of the National Health and Nutrition Examination Study 1999–2006 that assessed the cholesterol levels of 10,000 children ages six through seventeen.

According to a medical study in the '90s in Baltimore County, Maryland, 35 percent of America's school children have high cholesterol levels. This alarming fact was supported by the well-known Bogaloosa Heart Study in Bogaloosa, Louisiana, which concluded that 50 percent of the nation will die of heart disease if the current diets of schoolchildren remain the same. And Dr. Peter Kwiterovitch, founder of the Family Nutrition Education Program at Johns Hopkins Medical School, has stated that "proper diet could cut heart disease in America by 50 percent."

1. NUTRITIONAL THERAPY

Today it is widely known that food is capable of either causing disease or cultivating health. After such a long time in the closet, the medicinal qualities of food have finally begun to be recognized by Western science. Funded largely by governments and prestigious universities, more than 6,000 studies a year research the effects of various micronutrients in food. Ancient Chinese medicine and other alternative medicines that emphasize food as a primary healing therapy are no longer considered fringe therapies. Researchers have isolated a wide range of medicinal and preventive food properties that can eliminate or alleviate an extensive number of both chronic and acute diseases. On a cellular level, where all the action takes place, foods can act as anti-inflammatories, antibiotics, cancer fighters, cell insulators, cholesterol antagonists, hormone stimulators, laxatives, and relaxants, just to name a few.

It seems that almost every day newspaper headlines report a new study establishing the role of a particular food in the prevention or reversal of a disease. There are far-reaching implications in this research. Science is discovering the anti-cancer, antioxidant properties of cruciferous vegetables (broccoli, Brussels sprouts, cabbage, and cauliflower); the heart-healthy and other beneficial properties of various unsaturated fatty acids, including those found in coldwater fishes and raw, unprocessed olive oil, and most recently, the role of soybean products as protection against a variety of diseases, including a host of cancers and heart disease.

Soy has stirred a bit of controversy of late. I am constantly asked, in light of all the genetic modification of the soy crops, if soy is indeed healthy for men and women or those who have been diagnosed with estrogen-positive cancers. Soy contains 2.0 alpha hydroxyl esterone, the estrogen that is derived from plants. The animal-based 1.6 alpha hydroxyl esterone is formulated for use in hormone replacement therapy (HRT). Not all estrogens are created equal. The animal-based 1.6 is the controversial estrogen that has been implicated as a heart disease and cancer risk in study after study. Many studies point out that the 2.0 plant-based estrogen actually reduces the effects of the animal-based 1.6 estrogen and many of its risks.

Plant-based estrogens are 1/2,000th as concentrated as the animal-based ones, and soy is an isoflavone that has demonstrated the ability to lower dangerous estrogens, prevent certain cancers, and reduce the risks of heart disease by lowering bad LDL cholesterol and triglycerides, while raising good HDL cholesterol. When you consider that virtually all diseases, including cancer and heart disease, are inflammatory diseases, it is also important to consider the anti-inflammatory properties of the essential fatty acid alpha linolenic acid that is contained in soy. My two soy caveats are simply:

1. Go organic in order to avoid genetically modified soy, and

2. Make sure you are not allergic to soy prior to including it in your diet. An allergy to any given food will cancel out most of the medicinal properties.

The body is maintained by thousands of processes more intricate than science can fully grasp. The intelligence encoded in a single strand of DNA is too detailed for even the best computers to unravel in a lifetime. The human body is a wondrous organism whose many biological miracles are impossible without the right food.

Proteins

Proteins have a number of functions. After water, they are the body's most plentiful and fundamental substance. Proteins are the major building blocks that create muscles, tissues, blood, and the internal organs. Proteins insulate cells, protecting them from invasion by bacteria, germs, and viruses. They are also the basic ingredients of enzymes and antibodies—integral parts of the immune response. I think of proteins as the Department of Public Works—they do all the repair work of the body's basic infrastructure. When a cut finger needs to be healed, when the immune system needs to be replenished, when cells are damaged from a virus, it's protein that does the job. Without protein, you don't recover from allergies, fatigue, illness, jet-lag, or any biological wear and tear.

Carbohydrates

Carbohydrates, the second major nutritional building blocks, create glucose, or blood sugar, which acts as fuel for the cells. Carbohydrates provide the body's most basic energy. Without carbohydrates, you have no fuel to support movement.

I break this group down into two fundamental types of carbohydrates: *processed* carbohydrates, such as table sugars and commercial bakery products, and *unprocessed* carbohydrates, which include fruits, legumes, vegetables, whole grains, and the natural sugars found in fruit.

Then I further divide both processed and unprocessed carbohydrates into high-starch and low-starch groups. High-starch foods are those with a total caloric concentration of 30–100 percent starch. Most processed carbohydrates are high-starch foods.

Unprocessed carbohydrates include a large variety of both low-starch and high-starch foods. Low-starch foods are those whose total caloric concentrations are comprised of 0–30 percent starch.

The body reacts very differently to these two types of carbohydrates. High-starch carbohydrates enter into the blood the fastest, due to their high glucose (sugar) levels. This causes an increase in the production of the hormone insulin which, in turn, triggers the release of an enzyme called delta 5 desaturase that increases the absorption of arachidonic fatty acid. Arachidonic fatty acid then increases the circulation of another hormone called thromboxane A2, which increases the clotting factor of blood and causes vasoconstriction in the arteries.

Simply put, high-starch carbohydrates cause the body to store and maintain fat, thereby enhancing the risk for weight gain and the accumulation of excess fatty tissue. They also increase the risk for developing heart disease, especially arterially induced heart disease such as atherosclerosis, which is a narrowing of the arterial wall. Additionally, after high levels of insulin are released in the bloodstream, sugar levels drop dramatically. This extreme back and forth yo-yo action between high and low blood sugar can ultimately contribute to a variety of diseases, including hypoglycemia and diabetes.

Low-starch carbohydrates, on the other hand, have what I call a low-starch index, which means they convert into sugar slowly and efficiently. They include such unprocessed carbohydrates as asparagus, broccoli, cabbage, cauliflower, celery, green leafy vegetables, and zucchini. High-starch, unprocessed carbohydrates include such foods as bananas, carrots, corn, peas, plums, and potatoes.

I strongly recommend that low-starch, unprocessed carbohydrates form the largest part of your daily diet. Not only will they give you a balanced source of abundant energy, but they contain a host of healthy micronutrients and will not convert to fat as readily as high-starch carbohydrates.

Even so, low-starch, unprocessed carbohydrates aren't preferable for all people all the time. It is important to remember the bio-individuality of each and every person. While high-starch, unprocessed carbohydrates can be a problem for anyone who is overweight or has diabetes, they can be nourishing for other constitutional types.

Additionally, although a high-starch, unprocessed carbohydrate, such as a carrot, may have a starch (sugar) index as high as table sugar, its effect on the body is very different from table sugar's. This difference has to do with the fact that sugar is a highly processed, *dead* food, while a carrot is a *living* food. Living foods are packed with enzymes that are responsible for expediting a number of biological processes, ranging from digestion to immunity. Although sugar, a processed, high-starch carbo-hydrate, and carrots, *un*processed high-starch carbohydrates, have a sim-ilar starch composition, they are significantly different on the energetic level. Just as identical twins have the same DNA but different souls, processed or dead foods have a different energy from that of a living food, such as a carrot. Additionally, living foods typically contain other nutrients that help the body digest them, as well as all-important fiber that protects against many diseases, including cancers.

As a general rule, I recommend that people reduce or eliminate their use of both processed and high-starch carbohydrates and increase their intake of unprocessed and low-starch carbohydrates, especially those in the living category. (*See* Chapters 5 and 6 on the five constitutional types and food flavors for more on the energetic aspects of foods).

UNBLOCKING ANDREW'S ARTERIES

No single food element is more addictive than starch, and no nutritional restriction is more unpopular. However, overeating high-starch foods can become a very serious problem if not properly managed. As much as 50 percent of all heart disease originates here, yet this problem is almost universally unacknowledged.

One patient who comes to mind is a classic example of this. Andrew is an attorney from Boston who came to see me several years ago after having been medically diagnosed with arterial occlusions of 90 percent, 80 percent, and 60 percent in his three major arteries. Doctors were encouraging him to have open heart surgery. Desperate and confused, he told me that for the past six years he'd exercised vigorously for ninety minutes a day, several days a week. He went on to explain that he'd been a strict vegan, restricting all animal foods from his diet, for those same six years. He'd also cut out all fats (butters, oils, mayonnaise, dairy products) from his diet. How, he wondered, could his arteries be so blocked when he followed such a healthy diet and lifestyle?

After thoroughly evaluating Andrew, I found that his diet was loaded with starches. He was eating mostly healthy starches, such as brown rice, beans, and bagels, but all high starch nonetheless. It was obvious to me that his starch load was contributing to what was surely a high-insulin, high-fat-conversion problem. I told him how these starches don't start out as fat on the plate, but do convert to fat in the body—with the same potential dangers as any cholesterol.

I took Andrew off the high-starch foods and put him on a low-starch, low-fat, protein diet. This, along with some dramatic supplemental support, helped reverse his condition. Adding the proper oils (borage and flax oils), and having him reduce his stress levels (stress produces adrenaline, which also triggers insulin) also helped turn his situation around.

Fats

Fats are the least appreciated and understood essential building blocks of life.

Essential fat is a term used to refer to a large range of vegetable fats and oils. As a food, fat is stored by the body for future energy needs. It also insulates and protects all cells, helps in the assimilation of proteins, normalizes bodily fluids, and much more.

Fats are divided into two broad groups: *saturated* and *unsaturated.* Within each of these categories, there are many different types due to the fact that fats are comprised of long chains of fatty acids, which can take a variety of forms.

Saturated fats are among the principle contributors to heart disease and a variety of other degenerative illnesses. They are most commonly found in fatty meats, dairy products, and processed junk foods. LDL, or bad cholesterol, which has long been recognized as a major factor in arteriosclerosis, high blood pressure, and multiple sclerosis, is one type of saturated fat. LDL cholesterol is found only in animal products, such as butter, cream, and fatty meats.

Another type of highly saturated fat, called trans-saturated fatty acid, or *transfat,* is potentially even more damaging than LDL cholesterol. Transfats are created by artificially hydrogenating liquid oils to make them firmer, as is the case with margarine. They are also most commonly found in deep-fried foods, such as French fries and bakery products.

One 14-year study at Harvard School of Public Health, called the

Nurse's Health Study, involved 80,000 nurses and was reported in the *New England Journal of Medicine* in November of 1997. It found that each 5 percent increase in calories (of total daily calories) from saturated fat, such as that found in animal and diary products, produced a 17 percent increase in the risk of coronary heart disease. Basically, this was nothing particularly new in the annals of research on saturated fat and the risk of heart disease. What was very important, however, were the findings on transfat and *monounsaturated* fat. Each *2 percent* increase in calories (of total dietary calories) from transfat produced a *34 percent* increase in the risk of coronary heart disease.[1]

Additionally, each 5 percent increase in calories (of total dietary calories) from monounsaturated fat, found in olive oil and salmon, reduced the risk of coronary heart disease by 20 percent.

As this and other studies continue to establish, many *unsaturated* fats, called essential fatty acids (EFAs), may actually *reduce* the risk of heart disease, high blood pressure, multiple sclerosis, etc. These EFAs are divided into two types—*monounsaturated* and *polyunsaturated*—and both types of EFAs are found in vegetables and seafoods.

Among the healthiest EFAs are omega 3s, whose food sources include coldwater fish, such as salmon and tuna. Omega 3s are believed to be responsible for many beneficial activities, such as reducing blood-vessel constriction, blocking the cancer-causing and artery-blocking activities of free radicals, emulsifying fatty deposits in the blood, and lowering blood pressure. Omega 3s can also be found abundantly in flaxseeds and their oil.

Olive oil is another monounsaturated EFA that is especially good for the heart. Among its functions, it lowers blood levels of LDLs (low density lipoproteins), the bad cholesterol, while maintaining healthy levels of HDLs (high density lipoproteins), the good cholesterol. (LDL cholesterol blocks arteries, while HDL cholesterol breaks up the blockages, emulsifies them, and flushes them out of the body.) Because olive oil is also more stable than other unsaturated EFAs, I recommend its use as a general, all-around oil. It is important to remember to eat as much of your oil raw as you can, in order to preserve its health-giving qualities. EFAs also enhance immunity through their ability to thin the blood, expediting circulation and the transportation of oxygen throughout the system. Many researchers, most notably two-time Nobel Prize winner Johanna Budwig, believe that low oxygen levels in the blood—the result of a diet high in saturated fats—is the genesis of all disease.

It is very important to note that fats are volatile, vulnerable to high cooking temperatures and harmful manufacturing techniques, which can often render potentially good oil dangerous. When buying olive oil, make sure it is labeled as first cold-pressed, extra virgin. With canola oil, make sure that it is labeled as cold-pressed or expeller-pressed.

Many of fat's most significant properties come from its ability to convert into a group of hormonelike substances called *eicosanoids* that regulate virtually all cellular activities, including anti-inflammation, immuno-competency response, and blood clotting. *Prostaglandins* are the best known health-producing eicosanoids the body manufactures from EFAs. Prostaglandins are responsible for the production of enzymes that are catalysts for all vital processes. Prostaglandins are largely responsible for regulating *all* gland and organ functions, including circulatory health and energy production. They regulate proper immune function, inflammatory responses, vascular stability, blood clotting, and brain functions. When prostaglandins are out of balance, serious health problems will occur.

There are three categories of prostaglandins (PGEs):

- PGE_1 prostaglandins are derived from *linoleic acids,* or LAs (found in most fatty nuts and seeds, high-starch grains, legumes, fruits, and vegetables, as well as many animal products), and *gamma linolenic acids,* or GLAs (found in evening primrose oil, borage oil, and black currant seed oil).

- PGE_2 prostaglandins are derived from *arachidonic acids* or AAs, found in meats, dairy, eggs, and peanuts.

- PGE_3 prostaglandins are derived from *eicosapentaenoic acids,* or EPAs, as well as *docosahexaenoic acids* (DHAs), both found in fish.

These substances have a profound effect on your health. For example, if a person eats excesses of high-starch carbohydrates, such as brown rice, potatoes, and beans (as do many vegans), this might contribute to a potential deficiency of the delta 6 desaturase enzyme, and it is this enzyme which is responsible for converting linoleic acids into gamma linolenic acids. When this conversion does not occur, the risk of cancer, heart disease, and other serious illnesses is increased.

Even with its complex needs and interrelated systems, the human body has an amazing adaptability and can survive on a variety of diets. Denied the essential substances it needs over long periods of time, however, the body loses particular functions and develops weakness, chronic illness, or life-threatening disease.

People accept this as an inevitable part of life, but it *isn't* inevitable. You hear the reports about trans-saturated fatty acids and sugar but don't take them seriously, wondering how it could be so unhealthy when your parents have been eating sweets, saturated fats, processed flour products, and minimal quantities of fresh produce for as long as you can remember. They survived, didn't they? But this way of thinking overlooks the connection between their diets and the fact that they're also a generation collectively plagued by a variety of chronic illnesses and erroneously accepts these as a natural part of the aging process. Except for rare individuals, in today's Western world there are no models of the aged who are agile, healthy, and free of degenerative disease. The fact remains, however, that if not for the ancient ancestors, there'd be no pictures of the possibility of human beings living into old age with vibrant health.

How ironic it is to have such relative wealth and the choices that wealth bestows, and yet be hurt rather than helped by the circumstances.

Perhaps people can change the way they think about food. With escalating medical and insurance costs, along with a rise in chronic illnesses, Western medicine is beginning to acknowledge what its science has been exploring for the past few decades—that *food heals*. Perhaps this acknowledgment will help everyone learn more about the foods they eat and inspire them to take better care of themselves.

While there are basic dietary guidelines that can be of use to all people (*see* Chapter 14), an individual's needs are in a constant state of flux. Needs also change at different times in a person's life. I use the Chinese five constitutional types system to personalize the basic dietary guide-lines, thereby customizing food plans for individuals. To find out your particular type and the corresponding foods that are particularly good for you, refer to the questionnaire and Chapters 5–12 on the individual types: wood, fire, earth, metal, and water.

2. NATURAL MEDICINES

Natural medicines—both herbs and supplements—are the second main cultivators of life-force energy in this book, and I include them in several sections.

Supplements are concentrated foods, and as such, their use is indicated when a person needs more of a specific nutrient than the diet can provide. Vitamins and minerals perform hundreds of functions in the body without which you wouldn't be able to live. (*See* Chapter 16 and the last sections of Chapters 7–11 for specific uses of natural medicines.)

There is no doubt that supplements can be used as medicines to treat illnesses or enhance the health of a fit person in good condition. Researchers at the finest university medical centers continue to conduct vast and thorough studies on the effects of vitamins and minerals in reversing and alleviating degenerative diseases. Supplemental vitamins and minerals are used to prevent and combat a full range of conditions, including anemia, arthritis, atherosclerosis, free-radical damage, liver dysfunction, menopause symptoms, and prostate cancer, to name a few.

At the genetic level, all disease is the result of free-radical attacks on healthy cells. These attacks open the door for genetic expression of all hereditary disease factors via the myopathic pathways of expression. Antioxidants in foods and supplements represent the keys to our disease protection. As mutated free-radical molecules attack our healthy cells seeking to *vampire* their electrons, antioxidants such as vitamins A, B_1, C, E, and the minerals molybdenum, selenium, and zinc, are poised to donate electrons on our protective behalf. Antioxidants such as alpha lipoic acid go one better. They actually have the ability to convert the vampire radicals back into healthy antioxidants.

Each vitamin and mineral is known to perform a variety of cellular functions. When used medicinally, they can aid the body to regenerate, nourish, and detoxify various systems, organs, and processes.

By all accounts, every ancient culture since the beginning of time used remedies from the vegetable and herbal kingdoms. Every animal's instinct (including human's ancestors) is to seek out the balancing and restorative energies found in barks, grasses, roots, seeds, and weeds. From each botanical family, we find a magnitude of medicinal compounds. The family of iron plants, for instance, is rich in iron, while the family of lime plants has large stores of calcium, phosphorous, and potassium.

Originating in China, India, and Egypt, the formal use of herbal medicine is generally believed to date back some 5,000 years or more. The ancient Greeks, Romans, and Persians used herbal medicines, as did the Native Americans and South American Indians. The Amazon is still a rich source of medicinal plant compounds, containing some 300,000 species of plant life—the world *outside* Amazonia contains a total of only 50,000 species.

Today's science of nutrition has established that medicinal herbs contain at least twelve active substances that give them their healing properties.

- Besides vitamins and minerals, they are: enzymes, flavonoids, glycosides, mucilage, proteins, saponins, silicic acids, tannins/coumarins, trace elements, and volatile oils.

- Among their combined actions, they work as anti-bacterial and anti-viral agents, anti-inflammatories, blood purifiers, capillary strengtheners, cardiac stimulators, circulatory agents, connective tissue strengtheners, detoxifiers, expectorants, laxatives, and lubricants, to name a few.

Because so many people have become tired of the dangerous side effects of synthetic pharmaceutical drugs, there has been a resurgence of interest in herbal medicine. In ancestral times, there was little choice about which medicines to use, but today there is. You can pick and choose among variety of natural medicines, while also having the option of using pharmaceuticals, only when, and if, you must.

Many people use over-the-counter drugs, such as aspirin, ibuprofen, and other NSAIDS (non-steroidal anti-inflammatory drugs) on a daily basis without knowing they can be dangerous. In the U.S. alone, 33 million people spend 7.5 billion dollars a year on NSAIDS and 7,600 people die from their adverse affects, including liver toxicity. On the other hand, few people know that willow bark is an effective natural alternative to aspirin available in tablet form. White willow bark is good for headaches, inflammation, achy muscles, and joints. It's no surprise that several herbs have become very popular in both Europe and the U.S. in recent years, including ginkgo biloba. Ginkgo may be helpful for memory and for circulatory and immune problems; St. Johns wort helps relieve mild depression, moodiness, and anxiety; and Black cohosh, which Native American tribes called squaw vine because it was so good for the squaws, is being widely used as an alternative to hormone replacement therapy for many menopausal women. The list goes on.

You can refer to Chapters 7–11 to see which natural medicines are especially suited to your unique needs. These chapters are based on the concept of bio-individuality—the tenet that individuals fall into one of several different constitutional types that each have a particular range of tendencies, strengths, weaknesses, and needs. To find out more about a certain medicine, you can also refer to Chapter 16, which takes a predominantly Western approach to the chemical and mechanical properties of particular supplements.

3. MIND/BODY BEHAVIORAL MEDICINE

The disciplines that directly cultivate the life force by unblocking energy from the unseen realms are what I refer to as *Mind/Body Medicine* and it is covered in Chapters 12 and 17. As I've stressed throughout this book, holistic medicine refers to those medical models that acknowledge imbalances in *both* the mind and the body when searching for the roots of disease. Holistic medicine, therefore, integrates a wide array of disciplines, including those that address the physical body directly and those that address the mental and emotional realms directly. These therapies are also used to reduce stress and expand consciousness. Among the mind/body techniques available today are many types of meditation, including meditations involving movement, such as breathwork, ta'i ch'i, visualization techniques, and yoga.

Classical Chinese medicine, perhaps the first holistic medical model in recorded history, is a guiding principle in my practice. Much of my mind/body medicine is an adaptation of their work and stresses the importance of integrating complementary opposites: minds and hearts; right and left brains; intellect and intuition. (*See* Chapter 17 for details, including the script for a visualization exercise of this integration. *See* Chapter 12 for short, powerful ta'i ch'i exercises to bring mind and body to a meditative state.)

PART 2

The Ancient East

4

The Five Energies

The ancient Chinese believed that all of Nature was connected in one vast web of life. When they looked at the world and everything in it—people, weather patterns, emotional expression, developing illnesses, or learning processes—they saw similar energies at work. They also knew their fortunes were closely linked with Nature's changes, and they developed highly sensitive instincts that helped them recognize even slight changes in their surroundings and circumstances.

To a much lesser extent, people in today's world also respond to Nature's movements, dressing warmly if it's cold, seeking shade when it's hot, darting between shelters if it's rainy. Activities are also planned around energetic changes in Nature. If it's dangerously humid, you might cancel a hike, take a brisk walk on a cool, sunny day, or stroll the beach slowly on a foggy fall morning.

Emotions are affected by Nature, too. Often, the first warm days of spring are so stimulating, it's hard to contain your enthusiasm for life. Winter, on the other hand, may make you feel just the opposite—quiet and subdued, ready to hunker down and sit tight during the long nights ahead.

The ancient Chinese defined and organized the energetic changes they saw in the universe by categorizing them. They used the symbols yin and yang as the simplest way to describe the continual transformation of energy that was evident in the world. Everywhere they looked—from night to day, full moon to new moon, empty stomach to full, or sad to happy—they saw the universe expanding and contracting, fluctuating back and forth between complementary opposites that they named yin and yang.

In addition to yin and yang, the Chinese also used a system based on five energies to categorize the stages of change they saw in the world around them. Any phenomenon that is described in terms of yin or yang can also be more precisely described using one of the five energies. They can be used to refer to the different stages of any process or phenomenon, including the seasons of the year, the times of day, and the phases of a person's life. For instance, while winter and summer can be categorized as yin and yang, respectively, five energies thinking further breaks down winter's yin energy into two parts—metal and water—and summer's yang energy into two parts—wood and fire. In the center is earth, which represents a balance point between the extremes of yin and yang.

While yin and yang represent the concept of the cycling of any two polar opposites in Nature, they also describe and define two distinct energetic states of being. Yin, which we used to describe winter's nature, can be used to describe anything or anyone whose energy is withdrawn, inward, contracted, consolidated, potential.

Yang, on the other hand, is used to describe things that are extroverted, expanded, in full outward bloom, like the flowers of summer.

To really grasp what yin and yang mean, it is essential to understand that yin and yang exist only in relationship to each other: they are two sides of the same coin, just as night is the other side of day. One is not possible without the other, and they transform into each other over and over again, just as summer gives way to winter year after year. Put another way, ice, an extreme yin energy, is bursting with yang potential: it has nowhere to go but to turn to water. When the pendulum reaches its extreme point, it swings in the other direction. Contained within one energy lies its opposite.

The five energies, then, describe different phases of change. Using the yearly cycle to illustrate this point, begin with wood. Seasonally, wood corresponds to spring, when the ice has just melted and the first sprouts and green growth are bursting up toward the sun after having been in a contracted, dormant state all winter. Wood takes many of its characteristics from the way Nature is at this time. It is planting time, both figuratively and literally. Wood characterizes anything that is fresh, new, enthusiastic, and original. It is a time of rebirth, a time to begin projects, to expand, to launch something new, to reach out. Wood symbolizes energy stretching, unfurling, awakening from a long rest.

Fire energy follows wood and completes what was begun in spring. Seasonally, fire corresponds with summer, when the sun is at its hottest and the days are long. The flowers and plants that were just beginning to sprout up and form buds in the wood phase are now in full flower and bloom. Fire represents extreme yang energy. It is the time to reach for your greatest potential, stretch your limits, expand your capacity. You can understand and recognize this energy in anything from the radiant and fiery personality of a person to the height of an argument, the passion of lovemaking, or the childbearing time in a woman's life.

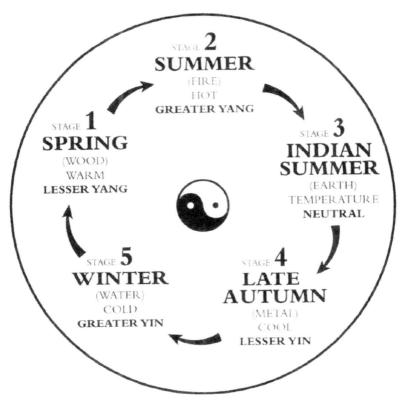

Seasons in a Circle.

Earth energy comes next. Seasonally, earth corresponds to late summer-early fall (or Indian summer), the time of ripening and harvest. This energetic phase is characterized by a brief period of balance and rest where neither yin nor yang dominates. It is still warm, but summertime is coming to an end. The days are beginning to shorten. There is still some outward activity, but harvest time means beginning to think about the winter ahead. Although the fire of the afternoon's sun is hot, there is a chill in the morning air. This is the earth phase, which represents an energetic state of being balanced between yin and yang. Earth characterizes anything that is in harmony, poised, and stable. Earth is the time to rest, to nurture, to unify, and enjoy.

Next comes metal. Seasonally, the metal energy corresponds to the fall. At this time, all of life is beginning to withdraw and turn inward. It's time to think about stocking up on supplies, stringing root crops in the basement, chopping wood for the winter. If you garden, it's time to put the garden to bed for the winter, pulling up the dead plants and turning the earth before it is frozen and can no longer be worked. Squirrels scamper across the fallen leaves, gathering nuts for winter. Metal is a time for reminiscing, reflecting, and analyzing what has gone before. It is a time for separating the wheat from the chaff, planning, and going inward. Metal can be used to describe a situation, person, time, or process that has these characteristics.

Finally, there is water energy. Seasonally, water corresponds to winter. In winter, energy has reached its most internal, hidden state. While there is little outward activity in winter, beneath the surface a lot is happening. It's a time of inner activity, internal fertility, and generation. Water restores and accumulates; it is extreme yin. Winter is a quiet, calm time when feelings run deep and everything awaits release. It's a time for strengthening, storing, and rebuilding the energy that has been spent.

As you become aware of the five energies, you will begin to see them at work in the world. Through this awareness you can start to recognize the subtle energies all around you. Seeing and defining these forces of Nature in yourself can help you find your connection to the greater whole and your place in the world. You are, indeed, a part of something bigger than yourself.

5

The Five Constitutional Types

Although you might like reishi mushrooms, I don't. In fact, they're not good for me, though they are undoubtedly good for some people. Similarly, while a midwinter visit to Arizona would be healing for one person in the middle of a cold and damp New England winter, it would aggravate the dry cough of another.

Everyone has a unique constitution with a whole set of different needs, tendencies, talents, and weaknesses. What is good for one person can be bad for another.

In Chinese medicine, the five constitutional types, an outgrowth of the five energies, are based on this idea. Similar to many other ancient healing systems, this system classifies people according to their different constitutions. Knowing your type—wood, fire, earth, metal, or water—will allow you to key into who you are inside and how you fit into the world. Knowing who you are in this system can help you focus on the kinds of foods, natural medicines, and inner changes that are best for you.

The use of the five constitutional types as a medical model for treating people according to their particular constitution is not unique to ancient Chinese medicine. Arabic medicine, classical Greek medicine, and India's ayurvedic system all held that there were different constitutional types of people. Perhaps the best known of these systems was the Arabic, which classified human beings into four types—sanguine, choleric, melancholic, and phlegmatic—that roughly correspond to the

Chinese types: wood, fire, metal, and water. The ancient Greeks, too, believed that all illness was merely the loss of life force that resulted from an imbalance in the fundamental elements: blood, phlegm, and yellow and black biles. And India's ayurvedic system distinguishes between three basic constitutions—vata, pitta, and kapha—that combine to produce ten possible individual types

The most fundamental principle of these systems is that human beings are cosmologically intertwined with Nature. Living in harmony with the natural world is considered essential for health and prosperity.

Chinese healers use the five energies to discover how their patients interact with the world. To do this, they have to take the time to probe all areas of the person's life—the physical, mental, emotional, and spiritual factors that reveal her or his individual energetic personality, or type.

Although individuals can be classified as one dominant single type, such as fire or water, more frequently people are a combination of two of the five types. For instance, a person can be a metal-water type or an earth-wood type. (*See* Chapter 6 and fill out the questionnaire to determine which type you are.)

Each of the five constitutional types represents functional processes fundamental to all human beings. While everyone has a particular constitutional type, people also have all the other types in less dominant roles. For instance, a fire type (someone with a strong will and fiery, passionate nature) may have earth characteristics when it comes to his or her mental capacities, or a love nature that is dominated by water characteristics.

Even though the desert is mostly dry, it also experiences, in various degrees, all the other weather conditions known on earth. This is how it is with people too. As you become familiar with the natural energies that the five types represent, you will learn more about the natural world, including the natural world within—human nature.

Everything you do reveals who you are. *You* adapt to things that come your way differently from someone else. How you process particular foods, store fat, metabolize carbohydrates, how you respond to angry words or react to various types of weather conditions, are all clues to *your* basic constitution. Knowing your type can guide both you and your therapist or doctor toward the foods, herbs, activities, stress-reduction techniques, and climates that are best for *you*. Knowing your mind/body type also helps you stay away from the things that weaken your basic nature. Being aware of your predisposition to various types of conditions—your weaknesses and strengths—allows you to adapt to your environment in a positive, health-giving manner.

Knowing your mind/body type helps you see yourself in an expanded way. Too often, the effect of society's one-size-fits-all thinking diminishes a person's sense of self. If you don't fit into the cultural ideal, you may judge yourself to be lacking. By becoming aware of the individual differences that the five constitutional types represent, you can begin to celebrate the spirit of connectedness and diversity that the ancients understood so well. By learning about your individual gifts and talents, you can begin to see yourself and others for who you *really* are and accept your individuality. Working with the five constitutional types can help you figure out who you are, why you're doing what you're doing, and what you can do to make the most of the gifts you have been given.

THE FIVE CONSTITUTIONAL TYPES AND CORRESPONDING INFLUENCES

The ancient Chinese were extremely knowledgeable about the natural forces in the world and the intricate ways in which they interacted with each other and human beings. This knowledge was consolidated and detailed in the five energies system. Each of the types corresponds to, or rules, an array of things and experiences. These correspondences include pernicious (damaging) influences, food flavors, emotions, bodily organs, times of the day, and so on. In fact, everything in the world can be said to correspond to one or another of the types.

The Five Constitutional Types and the Pernicious Influences

Each type is most vulnerable to one or more natural phenomena that have the potential to create illness. These phenomena are called pernicious influences and can result in a variety of symptoms, which will be explored in the following chapters on the individual constitutional types. It is important to grasp the general effect of these energetic influences, so you can learn to work with them.

The pernicious energetic influences arise as a result of either emotional, lifestyle, or environmental factors. Pernicious influences are classified as being either *internally* or *externally* generated.

The predominant pernicious *internal* influences are emotional-mental imbalances. Consistently repressing emotions or obsessively dwelling on them results in internally generated illnesses that can eventually create symptoms in the whole mind/body system, both internally and externally. (The emotions and their rulerships are explored later in this chapter.)

The externally/generated pernicious influences are a result of environmental and climate factors, including cold, dampness, dryness, fire, heat, and wind. For example, metal's dominant pernicious influence is dryness. This can be seen in the way metal types frequently tend toward dry coughs, dry, flaky skin, or maladies associated with a dryness of the internal organs. Because of this, metal needs to find ways to counteract dryness and create more dampness or moisture. Since this system of thinking is truly holistic, it follows that anything dry would worsen a dry condition. Therefore, metal types with dryness should avoid dry air, such as that produced by air conditioning or heating systems, dry climates, dry foods, and so on, and seek out its opposite, moisture, which will help balance it out and relieve the condition.

LAURA'S CUSTOMIZED HEALING FOR THE PERNICIOUS INFLUENCE OF DRYNESS

Laura came to me complaining that every autumn she got laryngitis no matter what she did. After a lengthy interview, we determined that she was a metal type. Metal is, of course, linked with the lungs, which are responsible for hydrating the body. Autumn weather, which is predominantly dry, is aggravating for a metal type. On an energetic level, Laura couldn't tolerate the added dryness to her already excessively dry nature, and she got sick every year at this time. I suggested some simple changes that would counteract all the dryness she was experiencing.

First, I suggested that she use a humidifier in her bedroom to moisten the air. I also recommended that she eat more vaporous foods—soups and stews—spend more time in the bath or shower, and take steam baths if she could, or spend time in the pool room at the local YWCA or health club. I suggested, too, that she stay away from pungent, spicy foods, which have a drying effect on excessive metal types. Instead, I suggested that she eat more of the sour food group, including barley, cabbage, citrus fruits, tofu, and yogurt, which all help the body hold onto moisture.

I also discovered that, while Laura's upper body was excessively dry, she tended to have a lot of yeast infections in her lower body, particularly in her intestines and vaginal areas, because she had excess moisture in her lower body. This energetic polarization of conditions often happens. The lower body becomes too damp, producing such symptoms as yeast infections or an edema (an abnormal accumulation of fluid beneath the skin), because the upper body is too dry. In Laura's case, the excessive dampness in her lower body was unfortunately an ideal condition in which for yeast to grow, just as algae grows in a stagnant pond. I knew we needed to get that lower-body moisture moving out and into her upper body. To do this, I suggested she stimulate the lower intestine by massaging it. I also encouraged her to release her repressed tears. All her life she had been the sad but stoic type, who rarely allowed herself to cry. But repressing grief causes an excess of overcharged drying energy to be stored in the lungs.

Laura was very willing to make these changes, and when she did, she stopped having laryngitis in the autumn.

In recognizing and counteracting the pernicious influences, it is important to remember the corresponding Chinese thinking: events and influences in the world (the macrocosm) correspond to events and influences in the little world or person (the microcosm). Thus, pernicious influences refer to the climate both inside and outside a person.

The pernicious influence of heat, for example, refers not only to high temperatures, but also to bad temper or hot flashes. Heat is also the condition of having too much activity, too much energy, in an area, whether it's in an organ, a section of the body, or an emotional-mental experience. By the same token, the pernicious influence of dampness not only refers to actual dampness, such as that found on a rainy or humid day, but also to excess mucus and phlegm in the body, and a lack of enthusiasm.

In Chinese medicine, good health in all the vital glands, organs, mind/body, and spirit is referred to as *harmony,* whereas disease is referred to as *disharmony.* Harmony and wellness are the result of balancing the subtle energies inside and outside of you. A healthy balance in all things is the key to wellness.

Here is a list of the pernicious influences and how they manifest in the environment, as well as the mind/body.

- **Wind.** Wind is active and is therefore seen as a yang phenomenon linked with the wood type and the spring season. Wind manifests gently in spring, hot in summer, cold in winter, and dry in the fall. The liver and spleen are most susceptible to the effects of wind. Except for the spring wind, which can be harmonious, wind is seen as the *most damaging* of the pernicious influences. It is characterized not only by wind outside in the world, but also by sudden change, often accompanied by a great sense of urgency. On the mental-emotional-spiritual levels, wind can manifest as sudden bad news, an abrupt encounter with rage or negativity, or a dramatic change in events. On the physical levels, wind manifests as sudden bacterial, germ, or viral infections, sudden bowel changes, allergic reactions, and breathing difficulties. Additional examples of wind include asthma attacks, convulsions, dizzy spells, fits of bronchitis, spasms, sudden fever, tremors, and twitches.

- **Fire.** Fire, both a major element and a pernicious influence, is an active, or yang, phenomenon associated with all the elements. It is characterized by the feeling or appearance of great heat. The heart and small intestines are most susceptible to the detrimental effects of fire. Characteristic examples of fire include boils, heat stroke, hot flashes, rashes, relentless determination, strong will, temper tantrums, and the personality of the type A workaholic. Fire often connotes an acute condition of some sort, whereas heat, which is similar to fire, is often indicative of a chronic excess condition.

- **Heat.** Heat is an active, or yang, influence often interchangeable with fire. Heart can manifest as damp heat in summer and dry heat in the autumn. The heart and small intestine are most susceptible to heat. It is important to note that heat can result from an excess of any of the other pernicious influences. An example of this would be a pneumonia created by exposure to cold and wind turning into heat—a fever.

- **Dampness.** Dampness is considered a yin phenomenon most commonly associated with the earth type and late summer. Like all the pernicious influences, dampness may manifest in any of the organ systems and may network its influence with other energies. The stomach and spleen, however, are most susceptible to its damaging effects. Dampness is characterized by a buildup of phlegm or mucus anywhere in the body, though it is most commonly seen in the lungs, lymph system, sinuses, spleen, and stomach, which causes colds, flu, viruses, and allergic reactions. Dampness is also characterized by frequent kidney, urinary tract, and yeast infections, as well as excess acid in the large intestine. Other characteristics of dampness include depression, chronic or acute fatigue, a diminished drive or desire, and a lack of emotional expression. Dampness tends to arise as a result of an energy stagnation in the lower body, with a corresponding energy excess in the upper body. For example, obsessive or compulsive thinking can pull excess mental or emotional energy to the head and upper body, leaving the lower body (bladder, intestines, kidneys, sex organs) damp and often cold from inactivity and stagnation.

- **Dryness.** Dryness is a yin phenomena linked with the metal type and the season of autumn. It is most often characterized by constipation, dehydrated skin, and excessive thirst. It may also be identified by pain in the lungs, or in the mid-thoracic and lower lumbar regions of the back. The lung and large intestine are most susceptible to the damaging effects of dryness. If gone untreated for a period, dryness will drain the ch'i (energy) from the kidneys, which are considered the body's reservoir. Therefore, those with excess dryness can have deficient kidney energy because the kidneys are responsible for cooling the body, and excessive dryness indirectly hampers the body's ability to stay cool. Since excessive heat is often a problem with the heart, it follows that dryness affects the heart's energetic equilibrium. You can see this is the way these pernicious influences move from one organ system to another. Therefore, excessive dryness can cause kidney deficiency, which can result in cold extremities, disc degeneration, frigidity, impotence, infertility, a lack of stamina, osteoporosis, and weaknesses of the lower spine.

- **Cold.** Cold is a yin phenomenon most often associated with the water type and the winter season. It is characterized by conditions that cause a profound chill or coldness to the body with a corresponding intolerance for cold. Just as it does in Nature, cold causes the body to contract, congeal, and slow down. The kidney and bladder are most susceptible to cold's effects, as it blocks the digestive and immunological flow of ch'i. Examples of cold include body aches, chills, lack of energy, poor circulation, slow movement, and even fever, which can be the body's attempt to balance the excessive cold influence. Cold can manifest as emotional distancing or aloofness. Excessive cold can result in the same set of symptoms as those associated with deficient kidney function, listed above under dryness.

The Five Energies/Constitutional Types and Corresponding Organs

The body's organs and functions are ruled by the five energies.

- The **fire** element rules the heart and small intestines. It governs warmth.

- The **wood** element rules the liver and gallbladder and governs glucose (energy), the muscles, ligaments, and tendons.

- The **earth** element rules the spleen and stomach and governs digestion. It distills food, converting food into blood.

- The **metal** element rules the lungs and the large intestines and governs vaporous hydration in the upper body. It also controls the filtration of air in the lungs and moisture in the intestines.

- The **water** element rules the kidneys and bladder, governing vaporous hydration, through the five fluids: digestive, hormonal, lymphatic, salivary, and urinary.

Chapters 7–11 have information on the five organ systems and the constitutional types with which they are linked. Each type is associated with both a yin and a yang organ, but this book focuses on the yin organ. (*See also* References in back for additional information.)

The Five Constitutional Types and Corresponding Food Flavors

As a nutritionist, I have used the five constitutional types extensively in relationship to the five food flavors, or food groups. This aspect of five energies therapy teaches that each human type benefits from one particular food group and is weakened by others. For example, the food flavor associated with metal is pungent, including such foods as garlic, leeks, onions, and scallions. These pungent foods are good for exhausted metal types since they are a vigorous food energy that, among other effects, improves circulation, including the circulation of moisture, which balances an exhausted metal type's tendency toward dryness.

The Five Constitutional Types and the Five Emotions

Emotions, too, are linked with the constitutional types. There are five basic emotions: joy, anger, sadness, fear, and compassion. Emotions are real energies that need to be expressed externally and, thus, released. If they're not fully realized and expressed, they store in specific organs as excess energy capable of negatively influence health.

For instance, unexpressed grief is stored in the lungs, and fear is stored in the kidneys. Since the body and mind work together, repressed emotion can often tip the balance and overburden a particular organ system, making it unable to cope with dietary excesses or other environmental stresses. I've had many, many clients whose ailments have been relieved when they began to acknowledge their grief, fear, or anger. Often, just telling them that emotions are legitimate energies that need to be expressed gives them permission to begin.

The Five Constitutional Types and Corresponding Emotions

- The **wood** type governs anger.

- The **fire** type governs joy.

- The **earth** type governs anxiety.

- The **metal** type governs grief.

- The **water** type governs fear.

Emotional pain needs to be understood in a more holistic context in this society. Painful emotions are not a bad thing, nor do they mean you've done something wrong or you're weak. They are simply an inner reflection of a part of your true self that must be acknowledged and experienced if you want to be whole and healthy. In other words, after darkness comes the light, after grief comes joy. When emotions are acknowledged, their energy is freed to move and transform, rather than remain lodged in the organs of the body.

The Five Constitutional Types as a Way to Find Balance

In simplest terms, this is about a system that sees life as a mixture of vital elements and seeks to balance them to promote health and healing. Too much or too little of anything upsets balance and results in illness. So, on a fundamental level, five-energies healing, as embodied in the five constitutional types, is a way to balance your individual blend of basic elements, including hot and cold, moist and dry, active and inactive, yin and yang.

Five energies thinking and the five constitutional types not only opens up the mind to the idea of balance in all things, but also to the concept of adaptability. Like the flexible willow tree that bends in the wind while the mighty oak gets felled, you, too, will do well to develop such adaptability to change. Knowing and accepting who you are gives you a deeper understanding of how you can artfully adapt to life and live more harmoniously with the natural forces all around you.

In the Chinese healing system, adaptability is the most desirable of all human qualities. To be able to embrace yourself and all things, rather than being contemptuous of what you're not or what has come your way, is a reflection of natural adaptability. To survive the inevitable losses and challenges that are an inevitable part of life on earth, you must be able to adapt. If you understand your energetic makeup—that you are particularly sensitive to cold, wind, or spicy food, or that fiery people make you feel anxious—then you can honor your constitutional uniqueness and take care of yourself accordingly.

6

What Constitutional Type Are You?

THE QUESTIONNAIRE

Although people are the same in many ways, they are also each very different with varying needs. Everyone is subject to the same array of influences—physically, emotionally, mentally, and spiritually—but each person responds differently.

Each one is unique. The diversity of the natural world is often masked by what seems, on the surface, to be the same. Working with the five constitutional types can help you distinguish who you are and how you are the same, or different, from others.

The following questionnaire is designed to determine your personal constitutional type and help you with your own customized healing. Your type doesn't change, it is a fundamental part of your makeup. People frequently discover that they are an equal mix of two of the five types, such as earth-water, or wood-metal, and in these cases, it is important to get to know each of the two types that define your constitution.

While each person has a dominant constitutional type, it is important to remember that not only is no one just one constitutional type, but each one is influenced by *all* the types to differing degrees.

The constitutional types represent varying ways of being in the world, and while a wood type will be largely extroverted and active, she or he will also have a deep, introspective water aspect somewhere within. Each person is made up of all of these energies, and it's important to recognize that their influence fluctuates. In one situation, you may feel, act, and react very much like your constitutional type, while on another day, or in another situation, you may feel, act, and react more like another type. These energies are all within you and they wax and wane.

This system of constitutional types is very useful when used simply or when probed more deeply to reveal a very intricate pattern inside you. It's helpful to realize, for instance, that you are a fire type who generates a great deal of excited energy that can easily exhaust you if not managed properly. It's most definitely useful for tailoring the basic dietary guidelines in Chapter 14 to your bio-individual needs.

You will come to understand how the different parts of your mind/body flow together and affect each other in an intricate tapestry that offers deep insight into your personal uniqueness as well as the nature of life itself.

Determining your principal constitutional type is extremely vital to becoming your own self-empowered healthcare manager. No matter what mix of conventional and complementary healthcare practitioners you may see, the ultimate responsibility for your health is your own. Knowing your primary constitutional type and acknowledging that people are all different are both first steps toward understanding the self. If you're going to be the doctor, you have to know the patient.

For each category, select the letter corresponding to the response that best describes you. For questions 1 and 4, please respond with an answer that best describes you during your formative and early adult years, even though you may no longer entirely fit that description.

RESPONSES TO THE QUESTIONNAIRE

You will most likely be a combination of types. The goal of this questionnaire is to find out your *dominant* type.

1. *Physique* (*In early adulthood*)   _____
   - (a) Square, well-defined frame
   - (b) Soft, round frame
   - (c) Broad, heavy frame
   - (d) Erect, medium build
   - (e) Thin, lean frame

2. *Weight*   _____
   - (a) Average to five pounds overweight
   - (b) Five to 10 pounds overweight
   - (c) More than 10 pounds overweight
   - (d) More than 10 pounds underweight
   - (e) Average to 5 pounds underweight

3. *Complexion*   _____
   - (a) Slightly oily, thick, and ruddy
   - (b) Very oily, burnt-brown tint, and red cheeks, dark
   - (c) Smooth, sensitive, hydrated, apricot tint
   - (d) Dry, thin, sallow
   - (e) Cold, clammy, pale white, thin skin

4. *Hair* (*Early adult years—your natural color*)   _____
   - (a) Moderately coarse, moderately thick texture
   - (b) Very coarse, extremely thick texture
   - (c) Wavy, medium texture
   - (d) Straight, thin texture
   - (e) Very straight, very thin texture

5. *Eyes*   _____

   (a) Focused, attentive

   (b) Distracted, expressive, intense

   (c) Warm compassionate

   (d) Piercing and penetrating

   (e) Deep reflective

6. *Appetite*   _____

   (a) Very strong at mealtime

   (b) Constant and strong

   (c) Moderate at mealtime

   (d) Light to moderate at mealtime

   (e) Little to none

7. *Elimination*   _____

   (a) Frequent constipation

   (b) Normal with occasional constipation under stress

   (c) Normal to slightly loose under duress

   (d) Vacillate between diarrhea and constipation

   (e) Frequent diarrhea

8. *Stamina*   _____

   (a) Good energy, good endurance

   (b) High energy, poor endurance

   (c) Moderate energy, erratic endurance

   (d) Low energy, poor endurance

   (e) Very low energy, very poor endurance

9. **Pulse** (*Resting*) _____

    (a) Quick and vibrant (70–80)

    (b) Fast and irregular (80+)

    (c) Moderate and even (60–70)

    (d) Slow and deep (50–60)

    (e) Very slow and shallow (40–50)

10. **Sleep Habits** _____

    (a) Light sleeper

    (b) Insomniac

    (c) Sound sleeper

    (d) Deep sleeper

    (e) Sleep disturbed by frequent urination

11. **Positive Mental Nature** (*At your best*) _____

    (a) Confident, independent

    (b) Enthusiastic, exciting

    (c) Supportive, caring

    (d) Logical, precise

    (e) Cautious, conservative

12. **Negative Mental Nature** (*At your worst*) _____

    (a) Obstinate, argumentative

    (b) Impulsive, consuming

    (c) Meddlesome, manipulative

    (d) Obsessive, ritualistic

    (e) Stagnant, unexciting

13. *Positive Emotional Nature* (*At your best*)   _____

    (a) Kind, giving

    (b) Joyous, optimistic

    (c) Compassionate, warm

    (d) Courageous, bold

    (e) Calm, peaceful

14. *Negative Emotional Nature* (*At your worst*)   _____

    (a) Angry, impatient

    (b) Vengeful, impulsive

    (c) Anxious, dysfunctional

    (d) Melancholy

    (e) Fearful, disassociated

15. *Spiritual Nature*   _____

    (a) Agnostic

    (b) Mystical

    (c) Pantheistic

    (d) Orthodox

    (e) Unorthodox

16. *Sexual Nature*   _____

    (a) Passionate

    (b) Magnetic

    (c) Passive

    (d) Dispassionate

    (e) Erotic

17. ***Your Persona In Family Relationships***   _____

    (a) Performer

    (b) Idealist

    (c) Peacemaker

    (d) Perfectionist

    (e) Escapist

18. ***Your Persona In Romantic Relationships***   _____

    (a) Loyal

    (b) Tempestuous

    (c) Warm

    (d) Detached

    (e) Mysterious

19. ***Your Persona Under Stress***   _____

    (a) Persistent

    (b) Burned out

    (c) Escapist

    (d) Intellectualizing

    (e) Avoiding

20. ***Affinity***   _____

    (a) To be independent

    (b) To feel pleasure

    (c) To feel secure

    (d) To have order

    (e) To be left alone

21. *Aversion*   _____

   (a) To be confined

   (b) To feel bored

   (c) To have to adapt to change

   (d) To be spontaneous

   (e) To be exposed

22. **Basic Instinct**   _____

   (a) To assert yourself

   (b) To attract others

   (c) To be caring and nurturing

   (d) To be organized

   (e) To persevere

23. **Life's Purpose**   _____

   (a) To make an impact

   (b) To be loved

   (c) To make peace

   (d) To implement systems

   (e) To teach

24. **Positive Archetype** (Your ideal image of yourself)   _____

   (a) The Spartan

   (b) The Charismatic

   (c) The Mediator

   (d) The Organizer

   (e) The Genius

25. *Negative Archetype* (Least desirable image) _____

    (a) The Intimidator

    (b) The Egotist

    (c) The Manipulator

    (d) The Perfectionist

    (e) The Recluse

MOST COMMON PHYSICAL SYMPTOMS

In each lettered column below, check only the most predominant symptoms/diagnoses that you have experienced, either acutely or chronically. Then total up the number of responses in each column; for example: 6 under *Category A* or 11 under *Category C,* and so forth.

Category A

Abdomen feels hard after eating	_____
Poor dietary discrimination	_____
Feel gassy after eating	_____
Crave fatty, heavy food	_____
Acne	_____
Dry, burning eyes	_____
Muscle cramps	_____
Tendonitis	_____
Labile hypertension (acute situations)	_____
Gallstones	_____
Conjunctivitis	_____
Hepatitis	_____
Glaucoma	_____
Menière's disease	_____
Migraine headaches	_____
Hormonal imbalances	_____

Otitis (earaches) _____
Impulsive, erratic behavior _____
Shingles _____
Mood swings _____
Light sensitivity _____
Blurred vision _____
Cysts _____
Endometriosis _____
Jaundice _____
Lead poisoning _____
Toxic pesticide exposure _____
Gout _____
Alcoholism _____
Drug intoxication _____

Total A Responses _____

Category B
Acute upper digestive heartburn _____
Eating too fast _____
Feel hot and sweaty after eating _____
Crave foods often and constantly _____
Red, burning ears _____
Fever blisters on tongue _____
Varicose veins _____
Rheumatoid arthritis _____
Essential hypertension _____
Raynaud's disease _____
Tachycardia _____
Hyperthyroidism _____
Heart arrhythmia _____
Parkinson's disease _____
Multiple sclerosis _____
Hot flashes _____

Mastitis _____

Nervous condition _____

Fainting spells _____

Hypoglycemia _____

Low blood pressure _____

Acidosis _____

Adrenal insufficiency _____

Cerebral Palsy _____

Hyperactivity (AD/HD) _____

Phlebitis _____

Tremors _____

Day sweats (overheating) _____

Blood clots _____

Hypochondria _____

Angina _____

Total B Responses _____

Category C

Excessive phlegm following meals _____

Sugar and/or starch addictions _____

Feel bloated after eating _____

Crave sweets and starch _____

Tender, bloody gums _____

Fever blisters in mouth _____

Stiff, aching muscles _____

Fibromyalgia _____

Colitis _____

Gastric or duodenal ulcers _____

Gastritis _____

Chronic fatigue viruses _____

Enteritis _____

Anemia _____

Hypothyroidism (underactive thyroid) _____

Prolapses (stomach, intestines, uterus) _____
Hemorrhoids _____
Diabetes _____
Nausea _____
Gum disease _____
Bruise easily _____
Parasitosis _____
Athlete's foot _____
Candidiasis (yeast infection) _____
Lyme disease _____
Pancreatic insufficiency _____
Mononucleosis _____
Anal fissures _____
Encephalopathy _____
Hodgkin's disease _____
Epstein-Barr virus _____

Total C Responses _____

Category D
Difficulty catching breath during meals _____
Dietary discipline (a fussy eater) _____
Nose, throat, sinus congestion after eating _____
Crave hot and spicy food _____
Bed sores _____
Loss of sense of smell _____
Pain with deep breath _____
Headaches with body aches _____
Asthma _____
Bronchitis _____
Emphysema _____
Sinus infections _____
Allergies _____

Cystic Fibrosis _____

Infrequent urination _____

Dehydration _____

Nasal polyps _____

Dry skin and hair _____

Sweaty palms and soles _____

Cold hands and feet _____

Sore throat _____

Strep throat _____

Tracheitis _____

Tonsillitis _____

Pharyngitis _____

Mastoiditis _____

Tuberculosis _____

Chronically inflamed adenoids _____

Appendicitis _____

Crohn's disease _____

Gingivitis _____

Total D Responses _____

Category E

Little or no interest in food _____

Always the last to finish a meal _____

Feel faint after eating _____

Crave salty or crunchy foods _____

Dark circles under the eyes _____

Loss of sense of hearing _____

Lower back pain _____

Osteoporosis _____

Kidney stones _____

Cystitis _____

Edema (fluid retention)   _____
Kidney/bladder infections   _____
Lupus   _____
Neprosis/Nephritis   _____
Sexual infertility/impotence   _____
Prostate disease   _____
Urinary incontinence   _____
Memory loss   _____
Insomnia   _____
Night sweats   _____
Sensory or motor difficulties   _____
Alkalosis   _____
Enuresis (bedwetting)   _____
Syphilis   _____
Anorexia   _____
Gonorrhea   _____
Scoliosis   _____
Mercury poisoning   _____
Bladder stones   _____
Agoraphobia   _____
Bulimia   _____

Total E Responses   _____

Now look at your total for each category. What lettered category (A, B, C, D, or E) has the highest total? The category letters correspond to the constitutional types below, so if the category with the highest total is A, then you're a wood type. If the highest total is B, then you're a fire type, and so on.

A. Wood   B. Fire   C. Earth   D. Metal   E. Water

7

Wood

Wood types are as exciting and impetuous as the first erratic bursts of warm weather in spring, as active as young children at play, as direct as the flight of an arrow. After the long confinement of winter, when all outside activity is at a low, spring bursts forth with an intense rash of expansive activity. Wood is linked with this season of rebirth and new beginnings. Just as spring fills the world with a riot of growth, so too are wood types eager to act, assert, and thrust themselves head-on into life.

Wood is a yang energy, which means it's active and expansive, focused on extending itself into the world. This is the opposite side of the cycle from the yin energy of fall and winter, when activity is concentrated beneath the surface and nature is quiet, restoring, and replenishing itself.

The wood type, then, is assertive and straightforward, as determined as the first green shoots bursting forth across dry and barren fields. Wood is full of creativity, resourceful at finding a way to make things happen. Wood types are enthusiastic and forceful, filled with a sense that a new opportunity is just around the corner. They're rough and rugged, strong, engaged and engaging, busy and involved. You don't have to wonder if a wood type is around, you'll always *know*.

Moreover, philosophizing and self-analysis is of little interest to this type. It's not enough for wood to believe in an idea intellectually without doing something about it. Wood types have a tremendous drive to establish themselves through action and are impatient unless they can move on their impulses. They're fast and determined, capable of accomplishing a great deal. No one is better able to initiate a project than the energetic wood type.

Wood types have a confident, positive attitude about whatever they do. They love independence and put great value on liberty and freedom. Wood types are honest, straightforward, and impulsive, so there is very little that is calculated or hidden about them. They are naturally outgoing, with a strong desire to stand out and be recognized for their achievements and their position in the community or environment in which they operate. Wood types strive to buck the odds, to be first at whatever they do. Much of their strength comes from their ability to persevere and work through whatever obstacles come their way. They have great willpower and good endurance.

Wood types tend to be adventurous, striking out to blaze their own paths. They're expansive, always testing their limits. They like the new and tend to gravitate toward innovative projects that others overlook. They are highly motivated and drive themselves hard.

Wood types can be self-confident, bold, and positive, but they can also be stubborn and argumentative. When wood types push themselves too far, they can spin out of control and become irritable and easily frustrated, lashing out in anger. They don't do well with sudden, unexpected circumstances or chaotic events because they have poor coping and adapting skills. Rather than finessing their way around obstacles they encounter, they tend to power their way through. Instead of stopping to pause and regroup, they charge ahead without thinking. While wood types can be great at getting a project off the ground, they can also become overbearing, not knowing when to quit. Too often wood types refuse to take the time to listen to others, they let their desire for immediate action get the better of them. If they are too impatient, they can scatter their energies and fail to complete the many tasks they have set for themselves.

Wood types are very active and forceful. They put out a lot of energy, but often their energy is so externally focused they don't take the time to eat well or take care of themselves. When they are exhausted and need to keep moving, they can unthinkingly become vulnerable to abusing food, stimulants, and alcohol. They live their lives with intensity, burning the candle at both ends, and are often the last to leave the party. Because of this, wood types frequently crash, burned out. This causes them to swing from extremely high to very low—they're either going 100 miles an hour or they stay in bed depressed all weekend. To feel best, wood types need to find a way to temper their extremist tendencies.

BASIC CHARACTERISTICS—
A SNAPSHOT OF THE WOOD TYPE

Wood types are generally of average to above average height with a square, athletic build and well-defined musculature. They are frequently five to ten pounds overweight, but rarely out of shape. Their complexions are often oily and thick-skinned, their hair thick and coarse. Their eyes reveal a direct, attentive stare, and they often have yellowish white.

They have a strong, hearty appetite and good endurance. Their pulse tends to be quick, bounding, and lively, with an average 70–80 beats per minute.

Their most common physical problems are vision and hearing impairment, headaches, high blood pressure, and elevated cholesterol.

Their positive mental attitude is confident, while their negative mental attitude is obstinate and argumentative. Emotionally, they can swing from being kind and giving to being angry. They have a natural affinity for independence and an aversion to confinement. It's their basic instinct to circulate and their purpose to make an impact.

WOOD AND THE BODY

The Wood Power Governs the Liver and Gallbladder

Just as the wood-type personality is great at getting things going in the outside world, the liver, with the adrenal cortex, is the organ responsible for getting things going in the mind/body.

The liver distributes energy throughout the body through anaerobic glycolysis, or the processing and combustion of glucose (sugar). In its role as the organ chiefly responsible for circulation, a healthy liver will supply the body with an even flow of blood and can both store and pump blood to ensure its even release.

The liver can be thought of literally as the live-er—the one who mobilizes life and vitality in the body. The Chinese refer to the liver as the *general* who is responsible for sending the troops (energy) around the body for vitality, filtration, and revitalization. As the regulator of the entire nervous system, the liver governs the functioning of the ligaments, muscles, tendons, and eyes.

When the wood type is firing smoothly and in balance, everything is flowing and circulating well, just as a healthy liver sends a balanced flow of energy throughout the mind/body. When the liver is healthy, it circulates, disperses, tones, and ventilates, keeping the system vital. It is the healthy inclination of both the liver and the wood type to circulate and move energy outward.

If the liver is impaired, circulation will be cramped. In the mind/body, this can cause little pockets of blocked emotional or mental activity; congested blood; fluid retention, or edema, especially in the face; and migrating inflammation and pain, which can result in elevated cholesterol. Because of the liver's role in storing and releasing blood, impaired liver function is also closely associated with menstrual and gynecological problems.

The functioning of the liver can be read by observing the condition of the fingertips and nails. Brittle nails and thin fingertips tell us that zinc absorption is deficient, or that a chronic virus has been present. It may also suggest that protein assimilation is inadequate due to protein enzyme deficiencies. Liver ch'i (energy) also opens up the eyes, so when the liver is healthy, the eyes read crystal clear. Conversely, if someone has yellowish or bloodshot eyes, this may reflect poor liver function.

Characteristic Wood Problems

Not all livers are healthy all the time, and not all wood types are healthy all the time. When wood types aren't able to channel their energy outwardly in an assertive, committed manner, they tend to draw their energy inward and become erratic, ambivalent, contrary, arrogant, and antagonistic. In this way, an unhealthy or out-of-balance liver impedes the flowing circulation of ch'i throughout the body. This lack of circulation and congested ch'i commonly causes an over-accumulation of dampness, heat, and wind in the wood type. These energetic imbalances, in turn, cause a variety of ailments, all of which are probable weaknesses and tendencies for the wood type.

While wood types exhibit good resistance to acute disorders, they're often riddled with chronic conditions. Commonly, these are a result of wood types tendencies to exhaust themselves by overindulging in excesses of all sorts, including emotional excesses, anger in particular. Since they tend to live life with such extravagance and intensity, they also tend to overdo everything, including their consumption of fats, sweets, spices, and alcohol, which leaves them depleted.

Wood can experience restless sleep and deficiencies in carbohydrate metabolism, such as low or high blood sugar. Alcohol addiction can also be a problem for wood.

Depending on the particular time, wood, like all the types, can either have an excess of high energy or an exhausted, low-energy state. These energetic swings are normal and affect everything in the natural world, including people.

When wood types are experiencing a period of exhaustion or low-energy, they are typically vulnerable to a range of maladies, such as blurred vision, chronic depression, cirrhosis, cystitis, diabetes, irritable bowel, low blood sugar, neck and shoulder tension, and sound and light sensitivity.

When wood types experience periods of high energy, they are typically vulnerable to a range of conditions, including boils, cholesterol elevation, connective tissue diseases, constipation, eye and ear illnesses, high blood pressure, inflammation of ligaments, muscles, or tendons, muscle cramps, and tinnitus.

A HEALING BALANCE FOR WOOD

Sour: Wood's Primary Medicinal Food Flavor

The sour food flavor is first drawn to the liver and gallbladder and is the most medicinal flavor for the wood type. Sour has a congealing effect that serves to bind or draw energy together. Perhaps the most specific conditions to benefit from sour foods are cirrhosis of the liver and other similar degenerative tissue problems. Much the way a lemon causes you to pucker your cheeks, sour's binding, gathering qualities help heal damaged tissue by drawing it together. In the same way, sour foods have a gathering effect mentally, and can help those with unfocused mental concentration. When wood types are exhausted and their energy is scattered and diffused, sour can help to pull them back to center and reenergize them. Sour is also excellent for diminishing the craving for sweets. Any weakened, sallow, emaciated, or melancholic, chronically fatigued conditions are especially helped by sour foods.

Examples of the Sour Food Group

Apple, barley, blackberry, blueberry, Brussels sprouts, cabbage, cherry, grape, grapefruit, hawthorne berry, kiwi, nectarine, orange, pear, pineapple, raspberry, scallions, soy, strawberry, tangerine, tomato, yogurt.

NATURAL MEDICINES FOR WOOD

Barberry Root Tincture

Barberry root is a bitter herbal medicine. The more bitter an herb is, the more cleansing it is. As the great naturopathic practitioner Dr. John Christopher once said, "The bitter, the better."

Its bitterness is due to a healing phytochemical called *ilicin*. Ilicin increases bile production in the liver/gallbladder region. This increases the alkalinity of the surrounding tissues since bile has a pH between 7.6 and 8.6. Every living environment has a pH, potential hydrogen factor: your houseplants, your grass in the backyard, your fish tank, even your swimming pool. The key to pH is that every living environment has a different requirement for homeostasis, or optimal balance. For optimal human health, blood pH should be 7.40–7.42, urine pH should be within the range of 6.40–6.80, and gallbladder pH 7.60–8.60. The higher the numbers, the more alkaline, the lower, the more acidic. In general, the lightly higher side of alkaline is considered healthier. Fruits, vegetables, and medicinal herbs are both alkaline and alkalizing. The more bitter herbs tend to be extremely alkaline, which triggers higher levels of bile salts. With the increased stimulation of bile, the liver is better able to return to an alkaline state, which allows the liver to do its job effectively—filtering out all of the accumulated toxins the body has ingested, such as food additives, pesticides, and certain fats.

Barberry is effective as a liver cleanser. I recommend this dose three times daily. Dissolve 10–15 drops in 3–5 ounces of pure water and sip on an empty stomach. Every six months, do this every day for one month. This is especially important for wood types who are careless with their diets.

Chrysanthemum Flower Tea (Chrysanthemum Morifolium)

The Chinese call this popular herbal medicine *jua hua* and commonly recommend that it be used as a tea. Generally, it's used to improve vision and relieve sore, tired eyes, but it's also often recommended for headaches associated with colds, flu, and allergies. Some studies in China suggest it is a useful herb for labile hypertension. Steep one tablespoon in a tea ball for 7–10 minutes to prepare a mug of tea. Drink 5–7 times a week.

Coenzyme Q₁₀

For the past thirty years, biomedical researchers have found hundreds of healing properties associated with this nutritional supplement. It has shown beneficial effects in treating a variety of conditions, including obesity and especially heart disease. And while it has even been discussed as a longevity enzyme in the *American Journal of Cardiology*, I prefer to use it as a liver detoxifier. It has a distinct ability to release liver/gallbladder pressure, and as a result it helps relieve associated symptoms, such as labile hypertension, sinus inflammation, migraine headaches, poor fat digestion, hormonal imbalance, irritability, and mood swings.

CoQ$_{10}$ was first isolated in 1957 by Frederick Crane, and in 1958 Dr. Carl Folkers first determined its chemical structure. It wasn't until the mid-'60s that Japanese researchers first discovered the CoQ$_{10}$ connection to congestive heart failure. This vital coenzyme is one of the keys to the body's production and distribution of adenosine triphosphate (ATP), or energy. The heart not only produces the highest amount of energy (5,000 times more electrical energy than the brain), it also requires the highest amount of energy. One of the all-but-forgotten issues relating to heart disease is the issue of heart energy. Heart disease isn't merely about cholesterol, it is about the replacement of all that generated, lost energy. CoQ$_{10}$ is essential for the replacement of heart energy.

Today there are more than 30,000 citations for the proven benefits of CoQ$_{10}$ in treating a wide variety of diseases, especially angina, arrhythmia, congestive heart failure, and high blood pressure.

Because statin drugs have been found to harmfully deplete CoQ$_{10}$ levels, it is important for anyone taking these drugs to replace it. Also, assimilation of CoQ$_{10}$ is often significantly depreciated in people over the age of forty, and those with a history and/or family history of heart disease tend to exhibit low tissue levels of this vital enzyme supplement as well. I recommend a dosage of one 200 mg capsule daily.

Holly—Bach Flower Remedy Tincture (Aquifoliaceae)

Like barberry, this is a superb liver tonic as it, too, is considered a bitter herb with high concentrations of ilicin. Interestingly, in its homeopathic form, holly is also a proven natural medicine for uncontrollable anger, rage, or temper tantrums. First formulated in the early 1930s by the British physician, Edward Bach, holly and the thirty-six other Bach flower remedies have been used successfully for decades by those seeking relief from a vast array of physical, emotional, and spiritual difficulties. I recommend sipping three drops in three ounces of water, three times a day, on an empty stomach.

5-HTP (5 Hydroxytryptophan)

This relatively new natural supplement has been described by many as Mother Nature's alternative to Prozac. 5-HTP dramatically improves the efficiency of the body's serotonin activity, which regulates the body's emotional state of mind and its sleep patterns. (This supplement should *not* be confused with the Japanese tryptophan that was recalled in the late 1980s because of a manufacturing flaw that was corrected.) 5-HTP is an over-the-counter supplement available at health food stores, and it can markedly improve sleep quality and mood stability, especially in the overstressed, overworked, excessive wood type. I recommend two 50 mg capsules daily on an empty stomach.

Linden Flower Tincture (Tiliaceae)

Over the centuries, linden flower has been used to treat a variety of illnesses. Among them are insomnia, nervous disorders, sinus headaches, and skin problems. In my work, I've found linden flower to be of great value in the treatment of various labile hypertensions, and I've seen great results with this natural medicine in many type-A personalities who have substantial wood factors. It has the ability to take some of the excess charge out of an overdriven nervous mind and body. I recommend fifteen drops in three ounces of water, three times a day on an empty stomach.

Natrum Sulphuricum (Sulphate of Sodium)

This homeopathic medicine is a preeminent liver and gallbladder remedy. It has been used over the years for a variety of health problems, including conjunctivitis, earaches, sinusitis, and even spinal meningitis. The remedy is a great value for wood types with acute sinusitis, chronic digestive gas, and hepatitis. I recommend a 6c potency. Dissolve three pellets under the tongue three times a day on an empty stomach for one month.

Choline (Liquid Chloride)

This supplement has been successfully used to enhance memory because of its proven ability to support brain-synapse communication. In my work, however, I most commonly use choline (a B vitamin) to reduce blood-fat levels (LDL or *bad* cholesterol and triglycerides). The high-living wood types who overconsume fatty, rich foods, alcohol, and sugars tend to do well with this natural supplement. Choline will also improve circulation, cardiovascular functioning, and memory. I recommend one teaspoon, three times a day with food. It also may be taken in juice.

S.O.D. (Super Oxide Dismutase)

The fifth most common protein in the human body, S.O.D. is believed to be an anti-aging enzyme that controls the balance between oxygen and the potentially dangerous free radicals. It aids the liver in its anti-inflammatory efforts and its detoxifying chores, and it also protects liver cells from free-radical damage and the dysfunctions caused by stress and poor diet. I recommend taking 1500 mcg twice daily with food.

Super Max EPA (Eicosapentaenoic Acid)

Eicosapentaenoic acid is what is called *good* cholesterol. Research has shown these fatty acids to be extremely effective in lowering *bad* cholesterol, but their medical value extends far beyond cholesterol reduction. I have found EPA to be irreplaceable in reversing many chronic inflammatory diseases, such as arthritis, fibromyalgia, and many forms of lupus. I recommend one 1,000 mg omega-3 fish oil capsule with meals three times daily.

JAY USES WOOD-TYPE REMEDIES TO RESTORE HIS HEALTH

I had been seeing Jay, predominantly a wood type, on and off for five years. A stockbroker in his late thirties, he had been a well-known college athlete, still played tennis, and was very active. Jay had a powerful, muscular build, and was slightly overweight. His personality was big— he was very outgoing and could, on occasion, be domineering. He was a real type-A personality—a high achiever, very dedicated to his work, intense, and fast-paced about everything.

When he first came to see me, he had chronic constipation and muscle cramps that kept him up at night. He also had boils and other skin problems, especially in the spring and summer, and there were some ligament problems from old sports injuries. Because he was drawn to very rich foods—sugar, red meat, cheeses—his cholesterol and triglyceride levels were on the high side.

I put Jay on a low-fat diet that centered on lightly steamed vegetables, lean proteins, and other vegetarian foods, such as legumes and tofu. I suggested that he narrow his variety of foods, reduce the volume of intake, and eat more fruits and vegetables during peak fire season, which is summer. I also stressed that he should eat bitter vegetables, such as asparagus, escarole, kale, or peas, which are very good for reducing inflammation and calming the nervous system. To accompany the diet, I put him on a variety of wood-type natural medicines, among them vitamins B_6, B_3, B_5, CoQ_{10}, choline and inositol, calcium, magnesium, and potassium. He also took linden flower to help lower his blood pressure and holly (Bach flower remedy) for his mental tension. All of these were recommended in standard dosages.

Quite soon after making these dietary changes, Jay lost about fifteen pounds with relative ease. His blood pressure decreased significantly, as did his cholesterol levels, which went from the high 200s down to just over 200. His triglycerides, which had been consistently hovering at 130–140 mg/dl. when we first met, decreased to around 80 mg/dl. His skin problems cleared up, and he is now much less bothered by cramping and pain from the old ligament injuries.

WOOD BREAKFAST #1

Scrambled Tofu with Soy Links

1 lb. firm tofu

$^1/_2$ tsp. olive oil

1 small leek, diced

2 scallions, sliced $^1/_4$" thick

Juice from 1 lime

$^1/_2$ tsp. turmeric

Mash tofu with a fork and add turmeric. Mix well. Warm oil on medium heat and sauté leeks and scallions until soft. Stir in tofu and lime juice, and cook over low heat 3–5 minutes. Serve with lean tofu link sausages.

WOOD BREAKFAST #2

Warm and Fruity Salad

1 red or green apple, chopped

$^3/_4$ cup organic strawberries, halved

$^1/_2$ cup seedless red or green grapes

$^1/_2$ cup blueberries

$^1/_2$ cup raspberries or blackberries

$^1/_4$ cup rice syrup or barley malt

1$^1/_2$ cups soy yogurt

Combine apple, $^1/_2$ cup strawberries, grapes, blueberries, and either raspberries or blackberries. Purée $^1/_4$ cup strawberries, rice syrup, and soy yogurt to make a dressing. Stir as much dressing as desired into fruit and mix well. Warm slightly.

WOOD BREAKFAST #3

Creamy Barley with Soy Milk

1 cup pearl barley

$3^1/_2$ cups vanilla soy milk

$^1/_4$ tsp. ground cinnamon

Add barley and cinnamon to soy milk in medium saucepan and bring to boil. Reduce heat, cover, and cook until liquid is absorbed, approximately 25 minutes.

WOOD LUNCH #1

Pepper-Lime Chicken

1 lb. free range chicken, cut into pieces

$^1/_2$ tsp. finely shredded organic lime peel

$^1/_4$ cup lime juice

1 tbsp. canola oil

1 tsp. freshly ground pepper

1 tsp. dried thyme

Broil chicken for 20 min. Stir together lime peel, lime juice, oil, pepper, and thyme. Brush chicken with lime glaze. Broil until cooked through and no longer pink.

WOOD LUNCH #2

Green Beans in a Spicy Yogurt Sauce

1 lb. green beans

3 tbsp. plain soy yogurt

$^3/_4$ tsp. ground mustard

1 tsp. arrowroot

$^3/_4$ tsp. ground cumin

1 tbsp. lemon or lime juice

3 tbsp. water

Steam beans for 10 min. Combine yogurt, ground mustard, arrowroot, cumin, and either lemon or lime juice. Add 3 tbsp. water and mix well. Add yogurt mixture to beans and stir together. Simmer covered 15 min. on low heat.

WOOD LUNCH #3

Tomato Lentil Soup

$1^3/_4$ cups uncooked lentils

1 cup cabbage

1 cup leeks

1 tsp. olive oil

8 cups water or vegetable broth

1 lb. can of tomatoes, chopped or crushed

2 tbsp. Bragg's Amino Liquid

Rinse lentils well. Sauté cabbage and leeks in oil on medium heat until soft. Add broth or water, tomatoes, and lentils to pot and bring to a boil. Lower heat and simmer 45 minutes. Add Bragg's and continue cooking 15 min.

WOOD DINNER #1

Orange or Pineapple Chicken

1 tbsp. Bragg's Amino Liquid

4 tbsp. orange juice or pineapple

2 tsp. arrowroot

$^1/_2$ tsp. finely shredded orange peel

2 whole med. chicken breasts

2 tbsp. olive oil

4 scallions, sliced into 1" pieces

1 tsp. barley malt, optional (if used it is added at the end)

1 orange, peeled and sectioned

Stir together Bragg's, orange juice, arrowroot, and orange peel. Cut chicken into 1" pieces. Add oil to a wok and cook on medium heat. Add scallions and stir-fry for 3 min. Add chicken to wok, stir-fry 2–3 min. Stir sauce and add to center of wok. Cook and stir until thick and bubbly. Stir in orange sections or pineapple chunks before serving.

WOOD DINNER #2

Beet and Carrot Salad

1 cup escarole

1 cup romaine

1 cup beets

1 cup carrots

1 cup celery

6 rings red onion

1 tbsp. olive oil

2 tsp. Molkoson (whey concentrate)

1 tsp. lemon juice

1 tsp. honey

Dash ground pepper

Combine all vegetables. Add dressing.

WOOD DINNER #3

Hawaiian Tofu and Vegetable Stir-Fry

1 lb. drained tofu

1 mixed cup of bean sprouts, broccoli,
Brussels sprouts, cabbage, kohlrabi, leeks, scallions, sliced thin

1 tbsp. olive oil

$1/4$ cup pineapple juice

1 tbsp. Bragg's Amino Liquid

2 garlic cloves, pressed

1 tsp. fresh ginger root

1 tsp. sesame oil

1–2 tsp. arrowroot

Slice tofu and vegetables into thin strips. Stir juice, Bragg's, garlic, ginger, sesame oil, and arrowroot together. Heat olive oil over med/high heat and cook vegetables. Add water if they start to stick. Add tofu and juice mixture and cook 2 additional minutes.

8

Fire

Fire is passionate, inspiring, and proud. Fire is linked with summer, when the sun reaches its most extreme point. The fulfillment of Nature's most extreme potential is seen in the fire type. The buds and seedlings that were sprouting in spring reach maturity in fire's season, and the world is filled with fruit and flowers.

Just as the sun is the center of life and everything revolves around it, fire types naturally take center stage. Fire personalities are the people who get excited about everything and are exciting to be around. Just as the sun penetrates into every nook and cranny on Earth, fire personalities radiate their consuming interest in life to everyone they encounter.

Fire types are very active and are yang in its most extreme. The fire type has an intense nature with a strong willpower. Passionate, creative, and emotionally energized, fire types don't sit in the corner quietly reading by themselves; they are externally focused. Fire types are hyperaware of their environment, so they are very affected by, and susceptible to, others, as well as intuitive about what others think and feel. Generous and openhearted, they constantly involve themselves with others. Since they're comfortable with people, they make friends easily. A fire type won't hesitate to offer advice to a perfect stranger or suggest what someone should do in a given situation. If a fire type hears you are going on a job interview, he/she will do everything in his/her power to help you prepare for it and pump you up with confidence. These types are almost always willing and able to respond to the needs of others.

Fire personalities live their lives with a strong emotional commitment and are very passionate about what they think and feel. They are easily moved by life and are open about their feelings. Where others might see something as mundane, fire sees all kinds of possibilities and exciting opportunities to explore. This quality, linked with fire's extraordinary ability to communicate, makes them charismatic leaders able to inspire others with a transcendent vision of life. Fire types are able to take the ordinary and make it seem extraordinary. Because of this, they often take leadership roles. They make great politicians, teachers, CEOs of companies, entertainers, and the types of salespeople who can sell ice in winter.

Fire types are enthusiastic, optimistic, confident, frank, and outspoken. They have good senses of humor and are playful and affectionate. Fire types are demonstrative and like to touch others—a fire type will pat you on the back, put an arm around your shoulder, or pinch your cheeks. Fire-type faces are very expressive, and their voices are loud as they hold forth in the center of a group.

While fire types are easy to have as friends, it can be hard for them to develop intimate relationships. They are idealistic and can be unrealistically romantic and distracted by images of ideal, unattainable love, while soulful, serious love can scare them off. It can be hard to be married to fire types because their attention is so easily caught by what is going on just over your shoulder or across the room. It is possible that fire types are unable to respond to the deep emotional needs of someone close, while at the same time they can get caught up in thinking about the greater good of society, or any group with which they are involved.

Although fire types have fertile imaginations and can dazzle the masses and sweep people away with their ideas and enthusiasm, less fiery personalities who don't understand that kind of passion may not entirely trust them.

"Is she for real?" some may wonder. "Is he speaking the truth? Coming from the heart?"

Fire types frequently tend to be type-A, high-stress achievers who never seem to slow down physically, mentally, or emotionally. They can be nervous and find it hard to relax. It is important for fire types to find an outlet to ventilate the excess energy they tend to accumulate. If they don't ventilate or cool off, they can easily build up too much internal heat. If, for instance, they have a mild upset on Monday and don't do anything about it, you can bet there will be another upset on Tuesday. By Wednesday, if they haven't expressed their anger or frustration, they are likely to blow up. When fire types build up too much energy like this, they can be overbearing. Where a wood type gets angry and impatient, fire can burn those around them with a blaze of rage that knows exactly where to strike to cause the greatest hurt.

BASIC CHARACTERISTICS—
A SNAPSHOT OF THE FIRE TYPE

Fire types are average to above-average height with soft, round frames and limited muscle definition. They are often ten or more pounds overweight. They frequently have coarse brown hair with reddish highlights and coarse, reddish skin. (When the ancients first established this system, they didn't know of any red-haired, freckled people, or they would have seen fire in them.) The eyes of the fire type are generally dark brown with pinkish whites. Their appetites are strong and constant, and their elimination is generally good, with only a mild tendency toward constipation.

Their energy is very high, but their endurance is poor—they burn out easily. Their pulse is fast and irregular, generally 80-plus beats per minute.

Their most common physical symptoms are cardiovascular problems: angina, atherosclerosis, elevated cholesterol, and heart disease.

Their positive mental nature is enthusiastic and exciting, and their negative mental nature is impulsive and consuming.

Their positive emotional nature is joyous and optimistic, while their negative emotional pole is vengeful and impulsive.

Fire types have an affinity for pleasure and an aversion to boredom. Their instinct is to consume and expand. Their life purpose is to attract love. Fire's positive archetype is the charismatic, their negative archetype, the egoist.

FIRE AND THE BODY

The fire energy rules the heart and small intestine. The heart is responsible for the movement of blood through the body's vessels; it regulates the blood vessels, arteries, capillaries, and blood-flow highway system. The heart works with the spleen to transform ch'i (energy) from food into blood. The heart houses the *shen,* or spirit, and the internal *joy body,* and it is responsible for igniting the spark of life. If the heart isn't storing a balanced amount of spirit, a whole range of mental-emotional-spiritual disorders can result.

The eyes are the window to the spirit; when someone is manic, depressed, or brokenhearted, it can be seen in the eyes. The ultimate visual diagnostic test for the heart is the complexion. If the skin has blue or purple tinges, this reveals stagnation in the arteries. If the complexion is red, rosy, or lustrous, it reflects a heart that is strong and healthy, with good blood circulation in the arteries and other vessels. The Chinese say that the tongue is the mirror of the heart, and that a pale or purple tongue tells you there is stagnant heart blood. If the tongue has an even red color, there is a good, balanced flow of blood through all the vessels.

Characteristic Fire Problems

Fire needs to burn, and the fire personalities must be plugged into projects and involvements so they can channel their intense, excessive energy. Their most damaging imbalances result from a tendency to accumulate the pernicious influences of heat and dampness, and fire types typically suffer from excitability and feverish conditions. They have creative minds that are usually overactive, and regardless of how they appear on the outside, their emotions are never far from being out of control. Fire types can easily accumulate excess amounts of energy in their minds, hearts, and bodies. They are similar to wood, but much more extreme. Typically, they are the type-A personalities who need to slow down and find some quiet time to restore and regenerate their inner resources.

Fire burns hot and then burns out. Once exhausted of their reserves, fire types can become depressed and disappointed. Fire types are so externally focused that when they are depleted and unable to sustain their energy, they tend to lose themselves in the people, places, and things around them.

Depending on changing conditions, fire types can swing from a high state of great excitement and expectation to a low of disappointment and unfulfilled potential that leaves them feeling impotent and defeated. Where they were once confident and bold, they can become weak and withdrawn. It is important for fire types to seek out periods of solitude to help them temper their tendency toward extreme excitement. A sense of self-awareness can guide fire types to finding a balanced approach to life that helps them stay the middle ground more of the time and neutralize their tendency to swing to extremes. Depending on the particular time, fire, like all the types, can have either an excess of high energy or be plunged into an exhausted, low-energy state. These energetic swings are normal and affect everything in the natural world, including people.

When fire types are in an exhausted, low-energy period, they are vulnerable to a range of maladies, including adrenal insufficiency; chronic fatigue; depression; dizzy spells; fainting; frequent chills; inability to concentrate; low blood pressure; pale, flushed cheeks; premature ejaculation; Reynaud's syndrome; and slow, irregular heart pulse.

When fire types are in a high-energy period, they can become vulnerable to the following conditions: atherosclerosis; bladder infections; burning, painful urination; cardiovascular disease; chest pain; cystitis; excessive perspiration; eczema; high cholesterol levels; irregular or rapid heartbeat; multiple sclerosis; Parkinson's disease; pulmonary hypertension; rheumatoid arthritis; and strong erratic pulse.

A HEALING BALANCE FOR FIRE

Bitter—Fire's Primary Medicinal Food Flavor

The bitter food group has special healing properties for all active (yang) types. It is particularly suited to the fire type. Bitter is the flavor capable of releasing excess heat from the body, reducing inflammation, settling down the nervous system, and drying water conditions, such as excess phlegm. Therefore, it can relieve hypertension, temper excess willpower, disperse fluid retention, and freshen foul breath.

Examples of the Bitter Food Group

Amaranth, arugula, asparagus, bean sprouts, beet greens, carrot tops, celery, chicory root, comfrey root, dandelion greens, escarole, globe artichoke, kale, mustard greens, okra, olive, papaya, peas, radish leaf, romaine lettuce, quinoa, rye, shellfish, turnip greens, watercress.

NATURAL MEDICINES FOR FIRE

Borage Oil

The prostaglandin action in borage oil (capsule form) has been shown to help regulate insulin levels, helping both hypoglycemia and diabetes. It has also demonstrated the ability to help many with hormonal imbalances, multiple sclerosis, obesity, and prostate inflammation. I have witnessed remarkable results when this substance is used therapeutically for hormonal problems in both men and women. I recommend 150–300 mg daily.

Calcium/Magnesium Citrate

Both calcium and magnesium perform many vital functions in the human body. Among them are cell-membrane permeability, energy production, blood clotting, and structural bone development. In fire types especially, nerve transmission and muscle relaxation are vital concerns. These two minerals calm highly stressed fire types, alkalize their acid-prone blood, aid in relaxation, and improve sleep patterns. I recommend 1000 mg calcium citrate and 500 mg magnesium citrate daily.

Flaxseeds

Flaxseeds contain an anti-inflammatory fat that often works well with borage oil at supporting general immunity. In this instance, it is better to take them in seed form rather than oil form to avoid the substance becoming rancid. However, bulk flaxseed oil is fine if freshness can be maintained. Nobel Prize–winning researcher Johanna Budwig lauds flaxseed as having anti-cancer, anti-cholesterol, and anti-arthritic effects. My work has enabled me to appreciate its heart-smart properties. It has consistently reversed dangerous cholesterol ratios while strengthening heart function, and I am convinced this is a result of reversing damage caused by free radicals. I recommend that all fire types take either 3 tbsp of seeds or 2 tbsp of oil per day.

Hawthorne Berry

This natural remedy has been used for a variety of ailments since the Middle Ages. The key active ingredients include bioflavonoids, such as quercitin and retin, as well as a host of proanthocyanidins. Its foremost use is as a cardiotonic and a relaxant. Studies indicate that it also has a balancing effect on blood pressure—lowering it when it is too high, and vice versa. This supplement has been shown to dilate blood vessels, thus increasing blood flow to the heart and its muscles. I use hawthorne berry (capsule form) as a cardiotonic and blood-pressure regulator and find it especially helpful for fire types who are out of balance. I recommend a dose of three 500 mg capsules per day taken on an empty stomach.

Impatiens (Impatiens Glandulifera)

This homeopathic Bach flower remedy is a proven stabilizer for any irritability and impatience accompanying severe stress. It is a perfect natural medicine for highly stressed fire types. I recommend 3 tsp in 3 ounces of water, three times a day on an empty stomach.

Kava Kava (Piper methystrum)

This natural medicine from the South Pacific is a proven, 3,000-year-old remedy for anxiety. A member of the pepper family, kava-kava root contains medicinal plant compounds called kavalactones, which are powerful muscle relaxants and lessen tension in the mind and body. I've found this most helpful for the highly anxious, panic-stricken fire type. I recommend, in capsule form, 500–750 mg per day on an empty stomach. (Caution: This natural medicine may cause drowsiness and should *never* be used with any prescription medications. If you feel drowsy while using kava kava, do *not* operate a vehicle or any other machinery).

L-Carnitine

This amino acid has consistently demonstrated the ability to dissolve bad cholesterol and other dangerous fatty arterial plaques. With fire type's tendency toward heart disease, L-carnitine is a natural medicine they respond to. It certainly gets my vote as *the* excess cholesterol terminator. I recommend 500 mg twice in the morning and twice again in the afternoon on an empty stomach.

Potassium Chelate

Along with magnesium, potassium is one of the supreme heart-smart nutrients. Nutritional science has established that potassium helps the body regulate both the heartbeat and blood pressure. Both the muscles and nerves of the heart are dependent on potassium for healthy functioning. Used with vitamin B_6, potassium is also a superior diuretic. I recommend 99 mg of potassium chelate in capsule form per day, and have found that fire types see superb results.

NADH (Nicotinamide Adenine Dinucleotide)

Also known as coenzyme-1, NADH is an antioxidant derived from proteins and vitamin B_3. Found in every cell in the human body, NADH increases the capacity of the cells to produce energy. It is one of the new supplement superstars that continue to show great promise in the area of healing the human nervous system. I am most excited about the research that suggests it may be of great potential healing value for many people with Parkinson's or Alzheimer's. These individuals and depleted fire types may consider supplementing their diet with 10 mg of NADH per day.

TMG (Trimethylglycine)

Trimethylglycine, TMG as it is often called, is a naturally occurring substance, a plant compound found most commonly in beets, broccoli, Brussels sprouts, and Swiss chard. A principal methyl donor, it has the ability to control homocysteine, a substance that many medical experts believe to be the number-one cause of a heart attack. Where previous research had indicated folic acid as the foremost antagonist of homocysteine, current research now shows that TMG is far superior. I recommend 300 mg daily with meals.

DIET AND SUPPLEMENTS ALLEVIATE DONALD'S PROBLEMS

Donald, predominantly a fire type, owns his own business. He is on the short side, overweight, and not very athletic. He is very outgoing, charismatic, and aggressive. He gets excited easily and is exciting to be around. He's very enthusiastic about life and uses a lot of hand gestures when he speaks. I've talked to a few of his employees, and they say that he is good at inspiring and motivating people.

When Donald first came to me, he was troubled by excess perspiration, which bothered and embarrassed him in public. He was also experiencing painful, burning urination, and we had very dry skin and eczema, which was worse in summer, fire's season. He was a classic case of excess fire.

I created a diet for him consisting of a lot of raw foods, primarily salads and fruits, especially in summer. I suggested that he eat more vegetarian foods in general, with a target range of around 75 percent of his diet coming from those sources. I took him off red meat and fatty dairy products and also suggested that he use a very low variety and volume of food.

To augment his diet, I put him on various vitamins and supplements: vitamin B_1 for his nervous system and type-A personality; B_6 for his urinary problems (he tends to retain water and B_6 is a natural diuretic); and the B vitamin inositol, a nerve tranquilizer that also has an emulsifying effect on fats. Additionally, I put him on choline to further emulsify fat and lower his high cholesterol and triglyceride levels, and potassium and magnesium to address some of his hypertension. I added the Bach flower remedy cherry plum and aloe vera juice for hydrating the skin and the bowel to relieve constipation.

Donald was very disciplined about his new regime, and all his symptoms cleared up considerably. He lost twenty pounds, and his physician took him off all his pharmaceutical medication. I now see him once a year for a checkup.

FIRE BREAKFAST #1

Minty Warm Amaranth

$1/2$ cup amaranth, rinsed and drained

1 carrot cut in half moons (slice horizontally down middle and slice thin)

$1^1/2$ cups spring water

1 spearmint herbal tea bag

Pat amaranth, carrot, and water in a medium pan over high heat and bring to boil. Add tea bag to mixture. Cover, reduce heat, and simmer 30–35 min. or until all liquid is absorbed and grain is creamy.

FIRE BREAKFAST #2

Pecan Rye Cereal

1 cup whole rye berries

2^1/$_2$ cups water

^{1}/$_2$ cup ground pecans

1 tbsp. rice syrup

Toast rye in 350°F oven for 10 min., then grind coarsely in blender. Bring water to boil and stir in rye. Add pecans. Reduce to low. Cover and simmer 30 minutes. Add rice syrup and serve warm.

FIRE BREAKFAST #3

Morning Quinoa Delight

1 cup quinoa

1 med. carrot, shredded

2 celery stalks, sliced

1 cup okra, sliced (optional)

2 cups water, vegetable broth, or chicken broth

1 tsp. turmeric

1 tbsp. water or olive oil

Rinse quinoa thoroughly to remove excess starch. Heat water or oil on medium heat. Add carrot, celery, and okra. Cook for 5 min. Add quinoa, water, or broth, and turmeric. Bring to boil. Cover and simmer for 15–20 min. or until water is absorbed.

FIRE LUNCH #1

Stir-Fried Shrimp with Quinoa

2 tbsp. water or olive oil

2 large carrots, sliced into matchsticks

1 bunch fresh asparagus, cut in 1" pieces

4 stalks celery, sliced

1 lb. farm-raised, shelled, shrimp, de-veined and rinsed

1 tsp. coriander

1 bunch watercress, rinsed and sliced into bite-sized pieces

Quinoa, cooked according to directions

Heat 1 tbsp. oil or water in wok. Stir-fry carrots for 5 min. or until tender. Add asparagus and steam with additional tbsp. of water until tender. Add celery, shrimp, and coriander. Stir fry for 3 minutes or until shrimp is cooked. Add watercress and serve over cooked quinoa.

FIRE LUNCH #2

Red Lentil Stew

1 cup red lentils, rinsed

3 carrots, chopped small

4 cups broth or water

$^1/_2$ dozen asparagus spears, chopped, or beet greens, cut into small pieces

1 lb. arugula or escarole

2 tsp. ground cumin

1 tbsp. fresh cilantro

Black pepper to taste

Simmer broth or water with red lentils and carrots for 30 min. Add asparagus, greens, and cumin, and simmer 10 min. Top with cilantro and pepper to taste.

FIRE LUNCH #3

Creamy Carrot Soup

$1^1/_2$ carrots, peeled and sliced

$^1/_2$ medium potato, peeled and sliced

4 cups vegetable stock

1 tsp. canola oil

$^1/_2$ medium onion, chopped

$^1/_2$–1 tbsp. finely chopped fresh ginger to taste

Dash of dry sherry

Dash of nutmeg

Chopped fresh parsley or cilantro

Put carrots and potato in a pot with stock. Bring to boil, cover, reduce heat, and boil gently until vegetables are tender, 30–45 min. Heat oil in skillet, add onion and ginger, and sauté, stirring, just until onion is clear. Remove from heat. When carrots and potatoes are tender, add onion and ginger to pot mixture and cook 5 min. on medium heat. Purée in blender. Flavor with sherry and nutmeg. Serve with parsley or cilantro.

FIRE DINNER #1

Brussels Sprouts and Orange Salad

1 tbsp. olive oil

2 tsp. Molkosan (whey concentrate)

3 tsp. orange juice

1 tsp. honey

1 tsp. ground ginger

1 tsp. grated orange rind

Dash of pepper

2 cups Brussels sprouts, halved

1 cup sliced fennel

2 small oranges, quartered

2 cups watercress

1 cup mesclun salad greens

Combine the first seven ingredients. Steam the Brussels sprouts for 10 minutes, then rinse under cold water. Combine all the ingredients. Toss well. Serve.

FIRE DINNER #2

Broiled Cod with Mustard Greens

4 oz. fresh cod

Ginger juice from grated ginger root

Canola oil

Bragg's Amino Liquid

Brush Bragg's on the fish. Rub oil and the juice from ginger onto the fish. Broil 10 min. per 1" thickness of fish, or until it flakes with fork.

Yellow Mustard Greens

1 tbsp. olive oil

1 medium onion, sliced

1 leek, sliced

1 bunch mustard greens,
chopped into small pieces

Turmeric

Bragg's Amino Liquid

Heat oil over medium heat. Add onion, leek, and sauté 2 min. Add greens and turmeric, and sauté 8 min. Add water if needed, and add Bragg to taste.

FIRE DINNER #3

Broccoli, Watercress, and Mandarin Orange Salad

2 cups broccoli florets

1 tbsp. olive oil

1 tsp. honey

2 tsp. orange juice

2 tsp. Molkosan (whey concentrate)

10 red onion rings

1 cup mandarin oranges, sliced

1 cup watercress

2 cups tossed greens

Dash of ground pepper

$1/2$ cup sliced almonds

Steam the broccoli 5–10 minutes. Rinse under cold water. Combine olive oil, honey, orange juice, and Molkosan. Add broccoli, onion, orange sections, and watercress to the sauce. Stir well. Spread over mixed greens, add pepper, and serve topped with sliced almonds.

9

Earth

E arth is as sure and solid as the ground beneath your feet, as nurturing as a loving mother, as sustaining as a vast field of corn, as sheltering as the walls of a house.

After the heat and fervent activity of the height of summer comes a time of effortless ripening. Late summer/early fall—the time of year linked with the earth type—is that in-between time of fulfillment and satisfaction. Earth represents this brief period of poise after the activity of summer, but before fall's harvest. This is the still point when the forces of day and night—yin and yang—are in perfect balance.

Earth is the only one of the five types that is neither predominantly yin nor yang, but is a blending of the two. Therefore, it is both active and withdrawn, both outward and inward, both expansive and contracting. Earth types, then, share this balanced energy. They are the peacemakers who like life best when everything is flowing smoothly. They are down to earth, cheerful, and pleasant to be around. They have an aversion to conflict and will do almost anything they can to keep events on an even keel. Earth types are driven to bring everything into the center, to unify opposing factions and create a nice, safe, secure environment.

Earth types are highly social and can be very relaxed and relaxing to be around. Through their love of people, earth types are able to instinctively identify with a wide range of people, drawing them in through a sense of shared values. In a group, they pull people together by focusing on what others have in common, rather than what divides them.

This attitude creates and sustains relationships that might have floundered without the earth type's intervention. They feel most secure in a large group of people who are working together cooperatively. It is very important for earth types to have a solid network of friends and family around them, and they're often the glue that holds a group together. They derive much security from this sense of connection to the world. Earth types crave security and feel for those who are without. Therefore, they're extremely compassionate and empathetic, always ready to lend a helping hand to those in need.

Earth types are grounded and practical, concerned that life's everyday needs be met for those they love as well as themselves. Home is the center of an earth type's world, and they love to share it. Food and making a home are a big part of their lives. They also do well working at home. If they do work at an outside office, their work space will be filled with warm, homey details. They need to have a warm, comfortable atmosphere around them as much as possible.

Earth types find their sense of place in the world through their placement in other people's lives and their need to be useful to others. They have highly developed protective natures and seek to extend their blanket of protection across their friends and family. Earth types do this by making things comfortable for others. They are the ones who send a container of food along to a new acquaintance, or offer to take care of the kids if you're busy, or make sure that your driveway has been plowed after a big snow storm. Earth types take care of earthly things and always try to make the world around them a comfortable place where things run smoothly. Unlike fire types, who take center stage, earth types control the action from behind the scenes.

Like all the constitutional types, earth types manifest their energies differently depending on whether they're at their best or not.

When their powerful need to keep their lives peaceful and harmonious gets out of hand, they tend to become very anxious. Sometimes, this can cause them to become manipulative and interfering as they attempt to control events and people. They are very concerned with security, safety, and being grounded, and this can lead to excessive worry when situations are in flux and events seem uncertain. Often, earth types will search outside themselves for something to help them calm their worries. This dynamic often accounts for the earth type's addictive nature, which can involve the overuse and abuse of any number of behaviors and substances, from food to drugs.

BASIC CHARACTERISTICS—
A SNAPSHOT OF THE EARTH TYPE

Earth types tend to have a round, thick frame and average height and weight. They have little muscle definition, though their flesh is firm. They have a soft, hydrated complexion that can tend to be the puffy. Their hair is often wavy with medium thickness and texture. Their eyes present a gaze that is inviting, warm, and compassionate. Their appetite is usually moderate and their elimination is normal to slightly loose. Earth types tend to have erratic energy, with moderate stamina, and endurance. They have an even pulse, generally between 60–70 beats per minute. Their most common illnesses often include swollen glands and chronic immune and digestive deficiencies.

Their positive mental nature is supportive and caring. Their negative mental nature is meddlesome and manipulative.

Emotionally, they can swing from being compassionate and warm to being anxious and perhaps even agoraphobic. Their affinity is for security; they are averse to adaptation and don't like change. Their instinct is to seek balance, and their purpose is to create peace. Their positive archetype is the mediator, and their negative archetype is the manipulator.

EARTH AND THE BODY

The earth energy governs the spleen and stomach.

The spleen is the primary organ responsible for digestion, which involves extracting nutrients from food, distilling them, and transforming them into blood. How well it does its job results in either a good or a poor quality of blood.

When the spleen's function is impaired, this leads to abdominal distention, edema (fluid retention), and fatigue. Spleen impairment also results in a burning stomach, candida, chronic viruses, loose bowels, a loss of immunological function, swollen glands, and tumors.

The spleen is the organ affected by worry and anxiety, so too much of these emotions will burden it.

A well-functioning spleen balances the mind. Food, through the functioning of the spleen, brings you *down to earth,* balances you chemically, and has an overall harmonizing effect. In Chinese medicine, peace of mind takes place in both the mind and the body and is reflected in the blood. And the spleen is responsible for transforming mental energy into a particular quality, or spirit, of blood.

Characteristic Earth Problems

Earth types have a moderately good appetite unless they are rundown or ill. They have a distinct affinity for sweets and carbohydrates, which can become a problem for them. When stressed, they're prone to overeat sweets and starches as a way to fill themselves up. While a small amount of sweet food has a harmonizing effect on the earth type, too much can be damaging.

It is essential to understand that the ancients had no processed sugars or sugar products, so to them *sweet* had a different meaning than it does today. Proteins, such as fish, meats, and poultry, were considered sweet due to their metaphorically sweet nature as commodities that were rare and precious. (*See* list of sweet foods in this chapter.)

A bit of sweet behavior goes far to soothe a troubled earth type.

The earth type needs to guard against the tendency to accumulate cold and dampness because these pernicious influences are potentially the most damaging for them. Mucus and phlegm, manifestations of dampness, can riddle the digestive system and the lymph glands. Edema, or fluid retention, another manifestation of dampness, is also a characteristic problem for the earth type.

Earth types have only moderately good resistance to chronic ailments, which tend to manifest as spleen, lymphatic, and general immune dysfunction. These problems can result in chronic fatigue, erratic appetite, frequent colds and flus, loose stools, and swollen glands. Earth types sleep soundly and need at least eight hours a night or they run down their immune systems. When not troubled by anxiety, they are usually early risers. At their most vulnerable, earth types can become easily depressed and disinterested in life. They may also be intolerant of many foods and highly sensitive to environmental conditions. Both their immune systems and their capacity to adapt to changing circumstances tend to be deficient.

Depending on the particular time, earth, like all the types, can have either an excess of high energy or an exhausted, low-energy state. These energetic swings are normal and affect everything in the natural world, including people.

When experiencing an exhausted, or low-energy period, earth types are vulnerable to a number of conditions, including acne, anemia, bloating, bloody gums, chronic allergies, chronic fatigue syndrome, cysts, hyperthyroidism, loose stools, lumps, multiple chemical sensitivity, slow wound healing, swollen tissue, tooth decay, tumors, uterine and stomach polyps, varicose veins, weak wrists and ankles, and yeast infections.

When earth types are experiencing a period of high energy, they can become vulnerable to a range of maladies, including conjunctivitis, leukemia, lymphatic cancer, mood swings, panic and anxiety, phlegmatic eyes, ears, nose, and throat, PMS, puffy eyelids, stomach cancer, sugar cravings, uncontrollable appetite, upper body sores, and water retention.

A HEALING BALANCE FOR EARTH

Sweet—Earth's Primary Medicinal Food Flavor

Limited, unconcentrated amounts of the sweet foods will energize earth types. This is especially true when they are in a low-energy, deficient period. In Chinese medicine, the sweet flavor (excluding processed sugars) aids the digestive processes, giving short-term strength to the stomach and spleen. Sweet can then both aid digestion and soothe the spirits, temporarily reversing anxiety, tension, and fatigue.

Examples of the Sweet Food Group

Almonds, apricots, avocados, bananas, bass, beans, beef, beets, broccoli, cashews, cauliflower, chicken, cod, corn, dairy, dates, figs, flounder, haddock, halibut, ham, honey, lamb, maple syrup, melons, millet, oats, peaches, pork, potatoes, quinoa, raisins, rice, rice syrup, salmon, sesame seeds, spinach, summer squash, sunflower seeds, sweet potatoes, swordfish, trout, tuna, turkey, walnuts, wheat, winter squash, zucchini.

Note: Certain protein foods, which are classified as sweet flavored, are better for some types than others. For example: fattier proteins, such as dark poultry, eggs, ham, lamb, pork, red meats, and whole-fat dairy products (cheeses, sour cream, whole milk, etc.) are best avoided by all active (yang) earth types, as well as all wood and fire types. Most of these animal proteins can be better utilized from time to time by most deficient (yin) earth types, as well as all metal and water types. If eating red meat, eat very lean cuts. If eating eggs, cook thoroughly to avoid salmonella food poisoning. Lean proteins such as fish, lean poultry, and tofu are best for active (yang) earth types and all wood and fire types. Fatty dairy foods are generally disadvantageous and should be eaten sparingly.

NATURAL MEDICINES FOR EARTH EXCESS

Astragalus Membranaceus (Leguininosae)

Also called ma huang by the Chinese, this is the oldest and most widely used herbal tonic in Chinese medicine. They use it to strengthen the pericardium, or *heart shield,* said to protect a person from all incoming negative energies, ranging from *bad vibes* to viruses. Astragalus has consistently proven itself as an immune tonic. In providing support to the circulation of lymph and the spleen, it strengthens the immune system, and it has demonstrated the ability to lessen both frequency and duration of colds, flus, and symptoms of allergies. I recommend 1,200 mg per day on an empty stomach.

Beta Carotene

This celebrated member of the carotenoid family has clearly established itself among the top substances for bolstering the immune system. Scientists have been enamored with beta carotene's pro-vitamin A activity, and they have acknowledged that it possesses an anti-tumor component. Extracted from food sources, such as acorn squash, carrots, and pumpkin, this orange-pigment concentrate has shown a great ability to strengthen the immune system against everything from the common cold to cancer. While recent research seems to suggest that some of its carotenoid family members (alpha carotene and lycopene) are even more powerful, I am still an avid supporter of beta carotene. I recommend 10,000 IU (international units) per day as a food supplement to all those fresh orange and red vegetables.

Chromium GTF (Glucose Tolerance Factor)

Most earth types have an affinity for sugars and sweet desserts. The mineral chromium has the reputation of being an appetite suppressant for sugar because it helps the pancreas regulate the release of insulin more efficiently. This sugar-regulating mineral is an especially potent energy modulator for most earth types. I recommend taking 200 mcg once daily with food at lunchtime.

Wild Siberian Ginseng (Analiaceae)

Ginseng is perhaps the most storied of all Chinese herbs. Its therapeutic benefits have been lauded for nearly 8,000 years. As a tonic, it is especially noted for its ability to increase stamina and resistance to stress and disease. Wild Siberian ginseng (also known as ciwugia) is considered one of the most effective of all ginseng tonics. In recent years, it has gained attention for its powerful energizing effect on members of the U.S. Olympic team. I recommend 100 mg of this supplement in capsule form twice a day on an empty stomach.

Pau D'Arco (Taheebo Lapacho)

This South American tree bark has anti-bacterial, anti-fungal, and anti-viral properties. Most typically it is recommended for its anti-yeast capabilities. Earth types have a strong tendency toward chronic candida yeast as a result of their over-consumption of sugar and starch. Thus, for most earth types, I recommend one cup of pau d'arco tea once a day.

Propolis

A bee resin collected from the poplar tree, this natural supplement gets my vote as the consummate immune tonic. According to history, propolis was once used by the ancient army of Sparta to increase their strength and stamina before entering into combat. Recent research has shown propolis's efficacy on an array of stubborn viruses and bacteria. I exclusively recommend a propolis form known as Nordisk because I've seen what it can do firsthand, especially for colds, flu, and allergy-prone earth types. I suggest one Nordisk propolis capsule per day on an empty stomach.

Red Clover (Trifolioum Pretense Leguminosae)

Red clover has been used for everything from skin conditions to spasmodic coughs. I have come to appreciate its ability to keep the spleen and lymph system clean. Earth types are generally phlegmatic and benefit from this pleasant tasting herb in tea form. I recommend one cup per day, and up to three cups for phlegm-producing allergies, colds, and flus.

Vitamin E (Gamma Tocopherol)

Vitamin E is a well-known antioxidant that aids in the synthesis of DNA, RNA, and red blood cells. It also insulates cell membranes, protecting them from bacteria, germs, viruses, and free-radical damage. I find it irreplaceable for most deficient earth types as an immunomodulator. I recommend 400 IU per day with food.

Vitamin B₁₂ (Methylcobalamin)

This vitamin helps the body synthesize DNA and red blood cells. Most importantly, for exhausted earth types, vitamin B_{12} helps with blood-deficient anemia and fatigue. I recommend 500 mcg of sublingual (under the tongue) B_{12} with food twice daily.

White Chestnut (Bach Flower Remedy)

This Bach homeopathic tincture is quite helpful for pensive earth types who are overtaxed, overstressed, and physically run down from the resulting mental overstimulation. White chestnut slows down the endless rotation of worrisome thoughts that wear down the body. Anxiety, insomnia, obsessive compulsion, and worry are all candidates for treatment with this tincture. I recommend 3 drops in 3 ounces of water three times per day on an empty stomach.

STRENGTHENING JANET'S IMMUNE SYSTEM

Janet, whom I would classify as an earth type, came to me with a series of immunological problems. She had swollen lymph glands, digestive problems, tooth decay, and bloody gums. She was a former smoker and had a chronic phlegmatic cough. She had sugar cravings and a tendency to overindulge in sweets, junk foods, and baked goods. She was also consistently overweight by ten to fifteen pounds, and her thyroid was underactive, despite her being on thyroid medication. Her metabolism was very slow, and she also had chronic yeast infections and bloating.

Janet was a very pleasant person, easy to be with. When we talked about her history, I learned that she had a difficult family life and saw that she was in a state of chronic stress because she was the one holding it all together.

I suggested that she begin to eat more cooked, warm, and dry foods. I thought it was important for her to have a bit more protein, such as baked fish and poultry, which are considered sweet foods and harmonizing for earth types. I also suggested she eat very lean red meat a couple of times a week since she had a tendency toward deficient levels of vitamin B_{12} and folic acid. I recommended that she eat more sweet root vegetables, such as acorn squash, carrots, parsnips, and yams. Additionally, I told her that pungent vegetables, including garlic, ginger, leeks, and onions, would be good for her. I wanted Janet to bake and broil much of her food for the dry quality that baking imparts. Since she needed a bit more fire, I suggested she also do some light sautéing with covered pans and that she limit the variety and volume of her foods.

I put her on the Bach flower remedies white chestnut to help relieve her acute anxiety and agrimony to bind her self-esteem. I also put her on chromium GTF and glutamine to help reduce her sugar cravings; digestive enzymes to help with bloating and gas; the homeopathic remedy pulsatilla; red clover tea for the swollen lymph tissue; vitamins A and E; and vitamin C for her bleeding gums.

Janet made a lot of progress. Her gums stopped bleeding, her lymph glands returned to normal, her chronic cough cleared up, she was sleeping well, and she stopped experiencing acute anxiety.

EARTH BREAKFAST #1

Muesli

$1^1/_2$ cups rolled oats

$1^1/_2$ cups spring water

1 tbsp. apple juice

2 tbsp. rice syrup

$1/_2$ cup dried apples, chopped

$1/_2$ cup dried pears, chopped

$1/_4$ cup currants

2 tbsp. slivered almonds, chopped

In a large bowl combine all ingredients. Chill in the refrigerator overnight. Stir well and serve.

EARTH BREAKFAST #2

Oatmeal Supreme

1 cup oatmeal

$1/2$ cup diced apples

3 tbsp. currants

3 tbsp. walnuts, chopped

$1/2$ tsp. cinnamon

$1/2$ tsp. nutmeg

Rice Dream, as needed

Cook oatmeal according to the directions. Add the apples and cook until soft. Sprinkle on the remaining ingredients.

EARTH BREAKFAST #3

Fruity Almond Cream of Rice

$1/4$ cup cream of rice

$1/2$ cup organic apple juice

$1/2$ cup spring water

2 tsp. rice syrup

1 tbsp. dried apples, diced

1 tbsp. currants

1 tbsp. toasted almonds, chopped

In a heavy saucepan, combine the first four ingredients and bring to a boil. Reduce the heat and stir frequently until thick. Remove from heat and put the cream of rice in a bowl. Sprinkle on the last three ingredients and serve.

EARTH LUNCH #1

Rice Pilaf with Almonds

2 tbsp. olive oil

1 cup onion, chopped

3 garlic cloves, minced

2 tbsp. fresh lemon juice

2 tbsp. Bragg's Amino Liquid

1 tsp. turmeric

$1/2$ cup fresh basil, chopped

$1/2$ cup fresh parsley, chopped

1 tsp. fresh thyme

2 cups brown rice, cooked according to directions

Sea salt and pepper to taste

$1/2$ cup of sliced almonds

Sauté onions and garlic in olive oil for 5 minutes. Stir in lemon juice, Bragg's, and turmeric. Add herbs and rice, and cook on low heat for 5 minutes. Garnish with almonds.

EARTH LUNCH #2

Winter Squash Soup

1 large acorn squash

1 tsp. butter

1 medium leek, chopped

1 tbsp. olive oil

$1^1/2$ tsp sage, chopped

Dash of pepper

$1/4$ tsp. ginger

$1/4$ tsp. chili powder

$1/4$ tsp. allspice

$1/4$ tsp. cinnamon

5 cups natural chicken broth

2 medium Granny Smith apples

Halve acorn squash and remove seeds. Just before putting in the oven, butter both halves and bake for 45 minutes at 375°F, then let cool. Sauté leeks in oil until soft, add spices and broth. Simmer for 10 minutes. Add chopped apples and cook until soft. Scoop out acorn squash and add to soup. Let simmer for 5 minutes. Place in blender, then serve hot.

EARTH LUNCH #3

Oat Burger

12 oz. ground turkey

$1/2$ cup onion

$1/2$ cup carrots, grated

$1/2$ cup red pepper, diced

$3/4$ oz. quick oats

Dash ground pepper

1 tbsp. Bragg's Amino Liquid

Combine all ingredients and press into patties. Broil until well done. Do *not* undercook turkey.

EARTH DINNER #1

Roasted Turkey Breast

2 turkey breasts, halved

1 cup natural chicken broth

1 medium onion, cut in wedges

1 tsp. thyme

1 tsp. rosemary

4 cloves of garlic, minced

1 tsp. lemon rind

$1/2$ tsp. fresh ground pepper

Place turkey in baking dish. Pour broth over turkey and place wedged onion around it. Sprinkle remaining ingredients over turkey. Bake at 325°F for 45 minutes. Do *not* undercook turkey.

EARTH DINNER #2

Haddock Bake

1 pound haddock fillet

1 tbsp. organic butter

Rosemary and thyme, to taste

1 tbsp. dry mustard

$1/4$ cup dry white organic wine

1 small onion, chopped

Combine spices and butter, then spread mixture over fillet. Place fillet in parchment bag. Pour in wine and place onions over fillet. Seal bag and bake at 350°F for 8 minutes on each side or until flaking.

EARTH DINNER #3

Root Vegetable Medley

1 cup carrots

1 cup turnips

1 cup parsnips

1 cup yams

$1/2$ cup onion

1 tbsp. olive oil

Sea salt and pepper to taste

2 tsp. of curry powder (or to taste)

$1/2$ tsp. parsley

Dice vegetables. Sauté with olive oil in large skillet until soft. Season with sea salt, pepper, and curry. Top with parsley before serving.

Metal

Metal is refined, discerning, precise, and disciplined.

Seasonally, metal corresponds to fall, that time of year when Nature's outward display fades and dies back. The first cold and cutting winds begin to blow as the Earth turns away from the sun and the nights begin to grow long. Nature is moving inward. Dead leaves and decayed plants fall to the ground to serve as fertilizer for next year's growth. Plants encapsulate their essence into seeds that will sleep away the winter to awaken in spring. The bright flowers, plants, and bushes melt back into the earth from which they came. Squirrels scurry across the ground, gathering stores for winter. At this time, there can be a sense of sadness and loss as all that was born in spring and grew in summer dies away once again.

Fall is the time to separate the wheat from the chaff. To take the best from the past and preserve it for the next round of birth and growth. To toss anything that isn't useful anymore and keep what is fall. Metal is a good time to take stock of resources and sort through all that has been created in the previous, active seasons. To organize experiences and set goals for the future. To withdraw from the furious activity that marked spring and summer and delve inward to replenish inner resources. It is a time of reminiscing and reflection.

Metal types, then, take many of their characteristics from the season with which they are linked. As such, they tend to be disciplined, organized, efficient, and structured. They're analytical and critical, often approaching things as though it were their job to report what's wrong with a situation. They have a refined sense of beauty and are idealistic at heart. Metal types are inwardly focused and have highly developed mental and spiritual natures. They are thoughtful and conscious about what they do, thinking carefully before they act.

Metal types are conscientious workers who have a strong attraction for order and control. Their excellent ability at scheduling and prioritizing makes them great managers. Because they're so good at breaking a problem or situation down into its component parts, they make great analysts and consultants. They are patient, precise, and detail-oriented. They are goal-setters, capable of getting a job done well in a sequenced, orderly fashion.

Metal types have a very refined nature and a reserved demeanor. They tend to be impeccable dressers, with equally impeccable personal habits. They are regal and noble, with a quiet confidence that comes from knowing who they are and what they're doing. They have good boundaries and are not thrown off center by what others think. They are not impulsive and outwardly passionate, but are moved by deep convictions based on the way they believe things should be. They have high principles and are often idealists. They are straight shooters who like predictability, consistency, and routine. If they become imbalanced with an excess of metal energy, they tend to become obsessive and compulsive. In this case, their natural inclination to be of service to others can turn into self-righteousness and criticism.

While they have a wonderful capacity for discipline, the flip side of this can be a perfectionism that leads to rigidity. They have a tendency to overwork because they feel comfortable within the structure of a job. Metal types tend to lack spontaneity in social situations and find it difficult to be casual and relaxed. Because of this, they sometimes appear to be emotionally aloof. It can also be difficult for them to be intimate with others. It's important for metal types to guard against becoming rigid in their thinking and in their bodies. It's also important that they learn to go with their intuitive and innovative impulses so they don't become robotic in their reliance on the status quo. Metal types are also inclined to be melancholic—their yin nature reflects their tendency to feel sad and withdrawn from the world.

BASIC CHARACTERISTICS—
A SNAPSHOT OF THE METAL TYPE

Metal types are generally shorter than average with a small to medium-sized frame. They have well-defined musculature and tend to be five to ten pounds underweight. They have dry complexions with thin skin that is often sallow. Typically, their hair has a high sheen that produces bright highlights. They often have intense, piercing eyes but may often have cloudy whites. Their appetites tend to be light to moderate, and they are very disciplined eaters. Their elimination vacillates between the two extremes of constipation and diarrhea. Their stamina is generally low, and their endurance is poor. Their typical diseases are of a respiratory nature, and it's common for them to have irritable bowel syndrome.

Their positive mental nature is logical, precise, and analytical.

Their negative mental nature is obsessive and rigid.

Emotionally, they can be either courageous and bold or melancholic and depressed. They have an affinity for order and an aversion to spontaneity.

Their instinct is to organize, and their life's purpose is to implement systems. Metal's positive archetype is the organizer, and the negative archetype is the perfectionist.

METAL AND THE BODY

Metal power governs the lung and the large intestine.

The lung is responsible for converting oxygen into ch'i (life-force energy). Respiration is a very critical life process, and a decreased lung function results in an impaired immune function, rendering the body vulnerable to all kinds of diseases as well as overall weakness, exhaustion, and shortness of breath. The lung is responsible for oxygenating the blood and balancing body temperature. The lung, in conjunction with the thyroid, is also responsible for keeping the lymph fluids clean, preventing such symptoms as chronic sinus and inner ear infections.

Additionally, one of the chief functions of the lungs is hydration, and they work closely with the kidneys to regulate moisture, therefore making the lung responsible for hydrating the skin and hair. Healthy lung functioning will ensure healthy fluid metabolism, whereas unhealthy lungs will lead to swelling and fluid retention, especially in the face and head. Impaired lung function can also lead to urinary retention.

Chinese medicine says that because the lung openings extend all the way up to the nose, you can learn much about lung functioning by observing the breath. An even flow of breath through both nostrils reflects good functioning lungs, whereas blockages and uneven breath indicates impaired function.

CHARACTERISTIC METAL PROBLEMS

Metal needs to cut—to cut to the point, cut the bull, and cut through the extraneous to the essential nature of an event, experience, or resource. Metal is driven to strip things down to an archetypal ideal. When metal types take this perfectionistic tendency too far, they can become dogmatic, hypocritical, and rigid. Often, if this tendency becomes extreme, they can become very closed-minded and unyielding. This can result in a rigidity in the body that affects their breathing, their elimination, and almost all of their body's systems. It is important that this type learn that their way *isn't* the *only* way to go. Metal types need to guard against having too narrow a focus.

Typically, metal types have imbalances that result from a tendency to accumulate dryness and an inability to regulate hydration and lubrication in the body. They tend to have respiratory disease and can become run down or depleted by either excessive or repressed emotional sadness.

Depending on the particular time, metal, like all the types, can experience either an excess of high energy or an exhausted, low-energy state. These energetic swings are normal and affect everything in the natural world, including people. When metal types are exhausted, they speak softly, or lack a desire to talk at all, their appetite is weak, their energy is low, and their spirits are lagging. During these times, they can develop a variety of conditions: asthma; constipation; dark, scanty urine; dry cough; dry and itchy hair or skin; fever; respiratory allergies of a dry nature; sinus headaches; sore throats; swollen tongue; or tight and stiff muscles.

When metal types are in a high-energy mode, they can become vulnerable to the a wide variety of health conditions: allergies of a wet nature with excessive white or yellow phlegm; breast cancer; bronchitis; Crohn's disease; chronic sinus infections; clammy hands and feet; colitis; cystic fibrosis; excessive perspiration; incontinence; lung cancer; obsessive-compulsive disorder; rectal/colon cancer; or shortness of breath.

A HEALING BALANCE FOR METAL

Pungent—Metal's Medicinal Food Flavor

All metal types have a special affinity for the pungent food group. Pungent is an extremely vigorous food energy that can improve circulation, dissolve fatty deposits, distribute moisture to dry lungs and sinuses, and dry up phlegmatic conditions in the lungs. It can also detoxify pathogens and wastes from the intestines, blood, and urinary tract. The pungent food group has the energy to help clear the lungs of long-standing depression and repressed grief.

Common Examples of the Pungent Food Group

Carrot, cayenne, cinnamon, currant, bok choy, daikon, garlic, ginger, leek, mustard greens, onion, oregano, parsley, radish, sardine, scallion, turnip, turmeric, white pepper.

NATURAL MEDICINES FOR METAL

Antimonium Tartaricum (Tartrate of Antimony and Potash)

This is a classic natural medicine for any respiratory illness that is accompanied by a non-productive rattling mucous cough; short, difficult breath; or a dry, painful cough. Asthma, bronchitis, colds, emphysema, and flu are all aided greatly by this medicine, especially when there is little expectoration. I recommend it be taken in a 30c potency for up to three weeks—three pellets under the tongue three times per day on an empty stomach.

Beta-1 3D Glucan

Extracted from the cell walls of baker's yeast, this powerful immune enhancer has an affinity for supporting immune-cell production in the body. Macrophages are immune cells that act like a super-powered vacuum cleaner, sweeping through the blood, swallowing up bacteria, germs, viruses, and other invaders. It has also demonstrated the ability to protect cells against harmful radiation and free-radical damage. In my work, beta-1 3d glucan has clearly proven its special effectiveness in helping most metal types with lung, lymph, and other general respiratory illnesses, both acute and chronic. I recommend 100 mg once a day taken on an empty stomach.

Fenugreek (Tigonella Foenugraecum)

This pleasant-tasting tea is superb for all respiratory illness where the predominant symptoms are a heavy wet phlegm and congestion. One of the oldest medicinal herbs on the planet, it has been successfully used to treat ulcers, as well as a variety of other inflammatory conditions of the stomach and intestines. For all metal types who have either acute or chronic digestive disorders, I recommend 1–3 cups of fenugreek tea per day.

Gorse (Ulex Europaeus)

Gorse, a homeopathic Bach flower remedy, is also appropriate for the metal type's mind and heart, as it is intended to help heal grief energy. Designated for sadness, despair, and hopelessness, especially after much pain and grief, gorse is a superb natural medicine for the psyche of most metal types, or for that matter, almost anyone experiencing those emotions. I recommend three drops dissolved in 3 ounces of water, thee times per day on an empty stomach.

L-Cysteine

This amino acid is a cell-membrane stabilizer that is a great lung and lymph protector against cigarette smoke and pollution. It has also been shown to stimulate the immune activity of white blood cells in response to disease. It also breaks down respiratory mucus resulting from allergies, diet, and infection. This lung and lymph tonic/cleanser is a superior natural medicine for all metal types. I recommend 500 mg twice a day on an empty stomach.

Mullein (Verbascum Thapsus)

For centuries, this tincture has calmed inflamed and irritated nerves, helping people with respiratory problems control coughs and coughing spasms. It has the ability to loosen phlegm and help clear it out of the respiratory tract. It also tones and cleanses the respiratory system and is equally medicinal for the throat, tonsils, and sinuses. It has even demonstrated the ability to shrink warts and small tumors. I recommend 10–15 drops of mullein tincture dissolved in 3 ounces of water, three times a day on an empty stomach.

Myrrh (Balsamodendron Myrrha)

Like mullein, myrrh is a superb respiratory purgative and tonic. The primary difference is that myrrh is more of an antiseptic for the mucous membranes of the lung and lymph systems. Myrrh also gives great strength to the stomach and small intestines, but I primarily recommend it as a superb natural medicine for all lung disorders, especially for most metal types. I recommend taking it in tincture form. Dissolve 10–15 drops in 3 ounces of warm or hot water three times a day on an empty stomach.

Spongia Tosta

This natural homeopathic medicine is indicated for a croupy, wet cough rooted deep in the chest. Good for an asthmatic cough that is worse in cold air, bronchial catarrh, and profuse expectoration, this is a superb medicine for most deficient metal types. I recommend a 30c potency, taken for three weeks. Dissolve 3 tablets under the tongue three times a day on a empty stomach.

Borage Oil (Borago Officinalis)

The prostaglandin action in borage oil (taken in capsule form) has been shown to help regulate insulin levels, helping both hypoglycemia and diabetes. It has also demonstrated the ability to help many with hormonal imbalances, multiple sclerosis, obesity, and prostate inflammation. I have witnessed remarkable results when this substance is used therapeutically for hormonal problems in both men and women. For metal types with general immunodeficiency problems, this is a valuable aid in treating respiratory problems. Its greatest feature for metal types, though, is its anti-inflammatory action, which makes it very effective for asthma and bronchial inflammations. I recommend 1000 mg capsules with food three times a day.

Zinc (Gluconate)

Zinc assists with all protein and DNA synthesis in the body. It furthermore supports the lungs with carbon dioxide detoxification and disease resistance. I've found it to be a great help with all respiratory problems, especially where there is significant inflammation accompanied by a high level of copper in the body tissue. I recommend 50 mg of zinc gluconate daily taken with food.

PATRICK'S RETURN TO GOOD HEALTH

Patrick is an entrepreneur in his midfifties. He's always dressed to the nines—very neat, prim, and proper.

When I first saw him, Patrick complained of dry hair and skin, tight, stiff muscles, constipation, and a chronic dry cough. As we progressed, I began to see undiagnosed rheumatoid arthritis. This dry, inflammatory response is often described by the Chinese as a fire condition that dehydrates and inflames the lungs, as well as the joints, muscles, skin, and hair, and is seen as fire invading metal. The lungs and large intestines—metal's corresponding organs—were struggling to moisturize and hydrate themselves. Metaphorically, they were not able to offset the ravages of fire.

Since Patrick wouldn't do well with hot and drying foods, I suggested that he refrain from eating pungent foods, such as garlic, leeks, onions, and scallions. He needed foods that would offset heat and dryness, while creating coolness and moisture. In keeping with this, I suggested that he eat raw foods (fruits and salads) along with lean proteins, including seafood. I also put Patrick on cod liver oil to hydrate his dry skin and on flax oil for his bowels. I suggested that he take the home-opathic remedy antimonium for his dry respiratory, allergy-type problems. I did extensive testing on him for allergies to determine what foods he was sensitive to and suggested that he eliminate those foods.

Patrick followed my advice and his recovery was dramatic.

DAVID'S OWN WORDS ABOUT HIS ECZEMA CLEARING UP

I'd been seeing a number of dermatologists for close to fifteen years. The problem was constant itching and dry peeling skin on my hands and face. I would itch, and I'd scratch it, and it would bleed. The dermatologists called it eczema. I finally found one doctor I thought I was satisfied with, and I stayed with him for about five years. He'd give me medicine, and it would clear up, but then just come back again. Finally, he gave up and sent me to a doctor in Boston, who sent me to another doctor who was supposedly an expert. I tried a bunch of treatments with him—ultraviolet light and various ointments and prescription drugs. Finally, he just said he didn't know what it was.

Then a friend of mine where I used to work recommended Dr. Mincolla and I went down and saw him and what a difference. Almost immediately. Even just from talking to him I felt a lot better. He looked me over and told me to stay away from red meat and dairy products. He found a few fruits I should stay away from most of the time—I could have them once in a while, just like I could have a hamburger every three months or so; that isn't going to bother me. I started using rice milk on cereal instead of regular milk, and there's an ice cream made out of rice I can use, too, if I want. He also put me on a bunch of herbs and vitamins. Every time I left his office, he would say, "Hey, this is no real problem." And this is after fifteen years of other doctors.

Almost immediately, I got relief, and that was it. It was amazing. Right now, my hands and face are totally clear, no more itching and scratching. I've been seeing Dr. Mincolla a couple times a year for about three years and everybody's happy—I mean the rest of my family. It had been kind of miserable for them, too.

So diet and vitamins and paying attention to what he recommended is what did it. I'm very satisfied. Couldn't be happier.

METAL BREAKFAST #1

Black Currant and Ginger Pears

5–6 firm ripe pears, peeled and sliced thin

$1^1/_2$ cups black currant juice

2 tsp. ginger root, finely chopped

2 tbs. arrowroot

$^1/_4$ cup cold water

Add juice, ginger, and pears to saucepan. Bring to a boil and simmer for 15 minutes, or until soft. Dilute arrowroot in water. Add to pears and stir until thick. Serve.

METAL BREAKFAST #2

Cinnamon Rice Pudding with Currants
1 cup rice milk
$1/4$–$1/3$ cup brown rice syrup
$1/2$ tsp. ground cinnamon or 2 cinnamon sticks
1 tsp. vanilla or maple extract
2 cups cooked short-grain brown rice
$1/3$–$1/2$ cup currants

Preheat oven to 350°F. Blend rice milk and rice syrup in blender. Add cinnamon and vanilla and blend again. Combine with cooked rice and add currants. Bake in 9x13 dish for 45 min.

METAL BREAKFAST #3

Eggless Omelet
1 lb. firm tofu
1 cup soy or rice milk
2 tbsp. olive oil
1 scallion, finely chopped
1 tsp. oil
$1/2$ cup bok choy, sliced thin
1 leek, sliced thin
$1/2$ med. onion, sliced thin
$1/2$ pepper, sliced thin
2 garlic cloves, pressed
1 cup mustard greens
Pepper to taste
Fresh parsley for garnish

Heat oven to 400°F. Drain tofu and crumble. Place tofu and soy or rice milk in blender and blend until smooth. Stir in scallion. Place in two pie baking plates and bake for 35 min. Meanwhile, heat 1 tbsp. oil in skillet. Add remaining ingredients and cook until tender. Add pepper and parsley to taste. Cover omelet with vegetable topping.

METAL LUNCH #1

Boston Baked Navy Beans

2 cups pre-soaked navy beans

5 cups water

$3/4$ med. onion, chopped

3 tbsp. Bragg's Amino Liquid

$1/2$ cup currants (optional)

1 tbsp. olive oil

$1/2$ cup rice syrup

1–2 tsp. dry mustard

1 tsp. ground ginger

$1/2$ tsp. garlic powder

Place beans and water in saucepan and cook on low heat for 45 min. Save cooking liquid. Preheat oven to 350°F. In dish or bean pot, mix beans, onions, Bragg's, oil, and currants. In a separate bowl, mix rice syrup, spices, and 2 cups of liquid from beans or water. Add to beans in pot. Bake covered for 1–3 hours. Add water if mixture gets too dry.

METAL LUNCH #2

Turkey Burgers or Meatballs over Rice

$^1/_2$ tsp.each: basil, celery seed, marjoram, oregano,
sage, tarragon, thyme (or any combination)

$^1/_4$ tsp. white pepper, cayenne or chili pepper,
garlic powder, ground ginger

1 tbsp. fresh parsley

$^1/_4$ cup onion, chopped fine

2 tbsp. brown rice or oat flour

1 lb. ground turkey breast

Paprika

Mix spices (except paprika) with flour and then with turkey. Form into burger or meatball shape and sprinkle paprika on top. Bake in 400°F oven for 15–20 min. Serve over brown rice, cooked according to directions.

Creamy Brown Gravy

2 tbsp. brown rice flour

2 tbsp. canola oil

$^1/_3$–$^2/_3$ cup vegetable or chicken broth

1 tbsp. onion powder

1 tsp. basil

$^1/_2$ tsp. garlic powder

$^1/_4$ tsp. oregano

1 tsp. dried parsley

Heat oil on medium and stir in flour until smooth. Slowly stir in broth and seasonings, then cook, stirring, until thick or to desired consistency.

METAL LUNCH #3

Cauliflower Bisque

1 tsp. olive oil

$^1/_2$ cup onions, sliced

2 garlic cloves

$^1/_2$ cup leeks, sliced

4 cups water or vegetable broth

Florets from 1 medium cauliflower

1 cup soy milk

$^1/_8$ tsp. pepper

$^1/_2$ cup soy flour for added protein and thickening

Bragg's Amino Liquid added to the liquid base for flavor

1 tbsp. fresh or 2 tsp. dried dill

Toasted walnuts

Heat oil and cook onion and leeks for 10 minutes. Add garlic and cook 1 more minute. Add broth, cauliflower, soy milk, and pepper, and simmer for 30–45 minutes. Blend with a hand blender or electric blender until creamy. Sprinkle with toasted walnuts and dill.

METAL DINNER #1

Black Bean Salad

1 tbsp. fresh cilantro, chopped

1 tsp. ground cumin

1 tsp. ground coriander

1 tsp. cayenne pepper

1 tbsp. lime or lemon juice

2 tbsp. olive oil

2 cups black beans

1 cup tomatoes, diced

$1^1/_2$ cups bell peppers, diced, red, yellow,
or green pepper, or a mix of any 2 or 3

1 cup brown rice, cooked according to directions.

In small bowl, combine cilantro, cumin, coriander, cayenne, lemon or lime juice, and olive oil. Stir in beans, tomatoes, peppers, and rice. Refrigerate until ready to serve.

METAL DINNER #2

Ginger Chicken

2 tsp. Bragg's Amino Liquid

1 tsp. fresh ginger root, grated

1 garlic clove, minced

(4) 4 oz. skinless chicken breasts

In small dish, combine Bragg's, ginger, and garlic. Add chicken and marinate for 3 hours. Broil on each side for 8–10 minutes.

METAL DINNER #3

Fish Stew

$^1/_2$ lb. fresh haddock, flounder, or scrod

1 lb. tofu cut in 1" cubes

4 slices ginger root

1 tsp. Bragg's Amino Liquid

1 stalk celery

2 scallions

1 cup vegetable or chicken broth

2 tbsp. fresh parsley, dill, or basil, chopped

2 tbsp. coriander

Place all but parsley and coriander in a pot and cover. Cook 30 min., or until fish flakes with a fork. Garnish with parsley and coriander.

Water

Water is deep, penetrating, yielding, and pervasive.

Water is linked with winter, the most yin, or inactive, season of the year. Nature has turned inward to regenerate itself in preparation for the new active cycle that will come with spring. It is as though the Earth is pregnant with gestating life forms sheltered in the deep womb of Nature.

With water, nature has reached its most extreme point of inwardly focused being. Water's nature is to yield, and through its ability to yield it is capable of transforming what appears to be unmoveable, just as a canyon can be created by the gentle meandering of a river across rock. The seemingly subtle action of water belies its incredible power.

Water types, then, are the least physically, outwardly active of the five types. They are the most introspective, the most sensitive, the most mentally and spiritually developed. But this doesn't mean they're not strong. Their strength lies in their connection with the inner worlds and the source of all being. Water types can be deep, brilliant thinkers. They are serious, perceptive, original, and doggedly determined to think things through. Enigmatic and unusual, they dance to the beat of a different drummer. Water types are interested in what lies beneath the surface. They are the philosophers who want to know why we exist, what we are, where we come from, and where we're going. Their function is to extract the deep meaning behind appearance.

Although water types are deeply emotional, they aren't good at small talk and don't do well in large social situations. They tend to be loners who frequently have a hard time connecting with the outside world, while at the same time they are acutely aware of their internal connection to the universe. If you do find a water type at a party, she/he will not be the center of a large and laughing crowd like the fire type, but sitting in one spot deep in conversation with someone.

Water types are thinkers rather than doers. They are visionaries who have unusual, offbeat thought, and they are very affected by the unconscious and the realm of dreams and intuitions. They tend to artistic and scholarly pursuits, often making art themselves. Frequently, they are wise beyond their years. They're voracious readers and typically highly educated, frequently self-taught. They are natural teachers, who teach what they learn.

It's very important for water types to maintain contact with others so they don't get isolated and frozen in their own little world, just as water turns to ice. If this extreme situation evolves, the water type can become very fearful and can feel lost and alone. Physically, this can manifest as frailty, low-energy, and poor endurance. When they go too far in this direction, they can become very despondent, fearful, paranoid, and suspicious.

But when their energy is flowing well, their creativity abounds. They can be way ahead of others with their brilliance at art, physics, and history. When they're not in a positive flow, however, their thoughts can get very ungrounded, strange, and fragmented.

Because of water's tendency to be withdrawn, they often find it hard to maintain a positive frame of mind, and they can become easily discouraged. At these times, they can lose touch with the world and with their own strength and self-sufficiency; they can lose concentration and have a hard time distinguishing between reality and unreality. This can overburden their immune systems, which often results in sudden and dramatic illness. More than any other type, water types must be diligent about taking care of themselves and remaining grounded in the material world. It's important for them to get plenty of quality rest and sleep to recharge themselves. Although it often seems as if they're hanging onto the physical world by a thin thread, they have a surprising resilience due to their spiritual strength, which frequently carries them through.

BASIC CHARACTERISTICS— A SNAPSHOT OF THE WATER TYPE

Water types tend to be on the short side, with thin, wiry frames and little muscular definition. Their weight is usually ten pounds or more under the average. Their skin tends to be pale and thin, and they often have dark circles under their eyes. Their hair is straight and thin and tends to turn prematurely gray or white. Their eyes are deep and intensely reflective, with clear, white irises. Their appetites range from low to very low. Their elimination is frequently loose, their stamina low, and their physical endurance poor. Their pulses are slow and shallow at approximately 40–50 beats per minute. The most characteristic diseases of the water type are genito-urinary, hormonal, and blood deficiencies.

Their positive mental nature is cautious and conservative, and their negative mental nature is stagnant. Emotionally, they can range from calm and peaceful to fearful and disassociated. They have an affinity for solitude and an aversion to exposure. Their instinct is to yield, and their life's purpose is to teach. Water's positive archetype is the genius and their negative archetype is the recluse.

WATER AND THE BODY

Water energy governs the kidney and bladder.

The kidneys are responsible for reproduction, growth, development, and the balancing of fluids. It is thought that our prenatal essence, or hereditary influences, are stored in the kidneys. The Chinese called this essence *jing* and believed it to be largely responsible for our constitutional strength. The kidneys are thought to be the gateway to all vitality. The kidney is also responsible for refining the essence we extract from food, especially ribonucleic acid, or protein.

Kidney impairment can result in impotence, learning disabilities, premature ejaculation, problems with growth, sexual disorders, and urinary infections.

In children, the kidneys are responsible for the development of good bone marrow, which is vital to the production of blood. If the marrow is impaired, the brain, the bones, and the spinal cord are all negatively affected and this can result in serious immune problems, such as blurred vision, impaired thinking, lower back pains, and tinnitus.

On the upper portion of the kidneys sit the adrenal glands, which are responsible for heat in the body. Because of this, the Chinese call them the lakes of fire. The lower kidney is the fluid balancer of the body and is called the lake of water, or the drainage ditch. The kidneys open up into the ears and manifest in the hair. Hearing problems indicate a deficient kidney function. Loss of hair, poor hair quality, and premature graying can reflect poor kidney function. Excess fear stores in the kidneys. Conversely, poor kidney function will show itself as fear, hypersensitivity, timidity, and weakness.

Characteristic Water Problems

It is water's nature to withdraw from the outside world and delve inward. In keeping with this, their mind/body energy tends to be withdrawn and less physically vital than that of the other types. While their emotions and mental activity run deep, their stamina runs low. They also tend toward overly active nervous systems. Depending on the particular time, water, like all the types, can either have an excess of high energy or be in an exhausted, low-energy state. These energetic swings are normal and affect everything in the natural world, including people.

When water types are experiencing a period of excessive high energy, they can become vulnerable to a wide range of conditions, including bladder and kidney stones, bone cancer, bone tumors, chronic bladder problems, deficient perspiration and urine, gum disease, hardening of the arteries, hypersensitive nervous reflex systems, hypertension, impotence, insomnia, kidney infections, nephritis, osteoarthritis, osteoporosis, super erratic behavior, uterine and prostate cancer, and vision headaches.

When water types are experiencing an exhausted, low-energy period, they can become vulnerable to another range of conditions, including anxiety, cold extremities, disc degeneration, excessive fears, frigidity, impotence, infertility, insecurity, lack of stamina, osteoporosis, weak or stiff lower spine, and in extreme cases, agoraphobia or fear of going out into the world.

A HEALING BALANCE FOR WATER

Salty—Water's Primary Medicinal Food Flavor

The salty food group is able to moisten and lubricate the lungs and intestines. It is also credited with the power to soften and dissolve lumps, tumors, and nodes. Salt foods are especially suited to the sick and inactive, and they are considered the primary food medicine for all water types. Salty foods are also credited with the power to neutralize anxiety, unfocused thinking, and poor concentration.

The salty food group should be strictly avoided by all those who are overweight, have high blood pressure, or diseases of the blood. All fire and wood types should also strictly avoid the salty food group.

Examples of the Salty Food Group

Arame, bibb lettuce, bluefish, chestnuts, collard greens, dulse, earth salt, grapes, hijiki, kelp, kombu, navy beans, nori, olive, parsley, pinto beans, red clover, sea salt, sorrel, spinach, Swiss chard.

NATURAL MEDICINES FOR WATER EXCESS

Cranberry (Juice)

Cranberries have chemical components that shield human urinary-tract cells from bacteria. Recent research suggests they can reduce the risk of bladder and kidney infection by as much as 40 percent. Considering that it takes 147 dried extract capsules to equal one eight-ounce glass of juice, I recommend three to five glasses of cranberry juice per week for those water types who are prone to kidney or bladder infections. I suggest you buy the less sugary brands that are blended with apple or another, less tart juice.

Eupatorium Parpureum (Queen of the Meadow—Homeopathic)

This age-old remedy is most helpful with deep, dull kidney pain, enlarged prostate, impotence, kidney or bladder infections, lower back pain, and sterility. It is an ideal natural medicine for depleted water types. I recommend a 30c potency, taken for three weeks. Dissolve 3 tablets under the tongue three times a day on an empty stomach.

Mimulus Guttatus (Bach Flower Remedy)

This tincture is a superb medicine for the chronic known fears and apprehensions that typically haunt the water type. It's also helpful with timidity and low self-esteem and for building self-assurance. I recommend 3 drops in 3 ounces of water three times per day on an empty stomach. Take it as needed, indefinitely.

Multi-Enzymes (with Betaine HCL and Ox Bile)

Water types classically have great difficulty filtering proteins and calciums from the diet, and this places great stress on the kidneys. Multi-enzymes containing HCL are especially designed to help in these areas of digestion by taking the burden off the kidneys. I recommend that one tablet be taken at mealtime unless there is a history of stomach ulcers, and that usage be discontinued if there is a burning sensation in the stomach. Never take these with light meals or a snack.

Raw Kidney (Freeze-Dried Bovine Tablets)

These bio-regulators are very powerful kidney tonics that were first popularized in the classic European health spas in the 1930s. Movie stars and heads of state would travel around the world for injections of these raw bovine tissues. Today, they are in the form of freeze dried pills available at your neighborhood health food stores. I recommend one 500 mg tablet per day taken with food for up to one month at a time.

Rhemmannia (Glutinosa)

This classic Chinese medicinal herb has been used as a kidney tonic for centuries. The unprocessed root, or *sangday* as the Chinese call it, is considered the most superior of all herbs as an alkalizer of the blood and fortifier of the kidneys. For women, it is also quite useful in treating menstrual irregularities and infertility. I recommend two 1000 mg capsules taken every day on an empty stomach.

Uva Ursi—Bearberry (Anctostaphylos)

This is useful for cystitis, nephritis, and urethritis. It's a reliable diuretic, astringent, and has urinary antiseptic properties. I recommend two 1000 mg capsules daily on an empty stomach.

Vitamin A (Retinol)

Vitamin A has long proven its usefulness for water types. It is responsible for sperm production, egg development, and mucous membrane formation. In the 1960s, Adelle Davis wrote about the great importance of vitamin A for keeping the kidneys clear of arterial protein and calcium plaques. I recommend 10,000 units per day.

Vitamin B$_2$ (Riboflavin)

Like vitamin A, vitamin B$_2$ is an antagonist to excessive boron (a mineral) and calcium deposits in the kidneys. Also like vitamin A, B$_2$ keeps sluggish, weak kidneys clean and clear. I recommend 50 mg with food twice a day.

Zinc

This remains the premier fertility supplement. Among its many functions, it helps with impotence, kidney disease, prostate inflammation, and sterility. Zinc is an essential core nutrient for all water types. I recommend 25 mg per day with food.

ANDREW'S CAREFULLY LAID-OUT PROGRAM RESTORES HIM TO EXCELLENT HEALTH

Andrew first came to see me when he was in his mid-thirties. He is approximately 5'8" and small-boned. Andrew was thin at the time of our first meeting, and yet his abdomen was distended—he had a potbelly from a buildup of fluid in his lower intestines. Andrew had a frail quality to him; his voice was soft and his presence was light, as opposed to being solid, grounded, earthy. His hair had begun to thin when he was only in his twenties, and he had a receding hairline. His eyes were very translucent blue, like water, very attractive, and the whites were very white. At the time of our first meeting, his skin had a bleached look about it.

Andrew complained about a variety of ailments, including frequent achiness in his Achilles tendon and heels, lower back pain, frequent cystitis, and chronic urinary problems. He had difficulty sustaining an erection and experienced premature ejaculation, which was very damaging to his male psyche. His overall stamina was low, he had difficulty performing tasks, was often ill, and frequently missed work. After compiling a history on Andrew, I determined that he was primarily a water constitutional type in a state of low energy.

Andrew was very interested in using natural therapies to overcome his problems. I recommended that he discontinue the use of raw foods and fruits, even in summer. I suggested that he eat more root vegetables, such as carrots, turnips, and parsnips. I also suggested that he increase his use of very lean, red meat to several times per week. He needed the B_{12}, iron, and folic acid from meat to bind him together and strengthen him, to bring some yang energy to his overly yin state. I recommended that he use pungent spices, such as onion powder, garlic, cayenne, and turmeric. I told him to drink two cups of wild Siberian ginseng tea every day—it's a powerful yang tonic. I suggested that he sauté much of his food in olive oil in a covered pan to increase its yang properties.

I put Andrew on two tablespoons per day of emulsified fish oil, a potent source of omega-3 essential fatty acids. He also began taking 10,000 units of vitamin A and two 250 mg raw kidney tablets daily, along with a multi-enzyme with each of his three meals to help him digest his food. Typically, water types don't digest protein very well, although they need *more* of it than other constitutional types. I also suggested that Andrew begin practicing ch'i gung exercises, which he did.

Andrew and I talked quite a bit about his childhood years and the fearful environment in which he had lived. We used visualization exercises in many sessions in order to create clear imagery of self-esteem and self-empowerment, which worked well for him.

Andrew made all these changes, and about six months after he first came to see me, he began to show marked improvement in many of his problem areas. Within four weeks, almost all of his symptoms were gone. He has to be quite strict with his diet. He can't indulge in sugars, fruit juices, fruits, or dairy products very much at all. His sexual life is normal and he rarely misses work anymore. His stamina is better, his urinary tract infections are all cleared up, and his lower back pain is all but gone. He is very pleased with his improvement, and I now see him only once a year for checkups.

WATER BREAKFAST #1

Brown Rice Muffins

2 cups brown rice flour

$^1/_2$ cup of almonds, ground

Egg substitute, equal to one egg

$^1/_4$ cup honey

1 tsp. vanilla extract

1 cup vanilla soy milk

2 tbsp. vegetable oil

Combine the dry ingredients. Separately, combine all the wet ingredients. Combine both mixtures in a large bowl. In muffin tin, fill each receptacle $^3/_4$ of the way and bake for 25–30 minutes at 350°F.

WATER BREAKFAST #2

French Toast

1 loaf of yeast-free sourdough bread

1 cup of vanilla soy milk

2 eggs or egg substitute

1 tsp. of almond extract

$^1/_2$ tsp. each of cinnamon,
nutmeg, and allspice

Combine the last four ingredients and mix well in a large bowl. Slice the bread and dip into the egg mixture. Place in a baking dish and bake for 20–30 min. at 350°F. Flip them after 10–15 min.

WATER BREAKFAST #3

Oat Flour Scones

$1^1/_2$ cups oat flour

3 tsp. baking powder

4 tsp. rice syrup

4 tbsp. dairy-free sour cream

4 tsp. vegetable oil

2 eggs or egg substitute

Mix the dry ingredients together. Then mix all the liquid ingredients together. Combine both mixtures and blend well. Drop rounded tablespoons of the batter onto a greased baking sheet. Bake for 15 min. at 350°F or until lightly brown.

WATER LUNCH #1

Salmon Kebobs

12 oz. salmon

2 tbsp. water

2 tbsp. Bragg's Amino Liquid

1 tbsp. lemon juice

1 tsp. onion, minced

1 tsp. garlic clove, minced

$1/2$ tsp. pepper

$1/2$ tsp. basil

1 medium zucchini, sliced

1 medium onion, sliced

Marinate salmon in the first 7 ingredients for two hours. Place salmon, onion, and zucchini on skewers and grill.

WATER LUNCH #2

Rosemary Roasted Potatoes

1 lb. of red bliss potatoes

1 tbsp. fresh rosemary

3 cloves garlic

2 tbsp. olive oil

1 tbsp. butter

Salt and pepper to taste

Sauté garlic in olive oil, butter, and rosemary until garlic is soft.

Dice potatoes and add to the oil and rosemary mixture in the skillet for approx. 10 minutes. Transfer all the ingredients to a baking dish and bake in oven preheated to 350°F for 40 minutes.

WATER LUNCH #2

Lemon Chicken

1 cup natural chicken broth

2 tbsp. lemon juice

2 skinned 8 oz. chicken breasts

2 tsp. olive oil

$1/3$ tsp. thyme

$1/2$ tsp. rosemary

$1/2$ tsp. tarragon

Dash pepper and garlic powder

Pour broth and lemon juice into small baking dish. Rub each chicken breast with oil and place in dish. Sprinkle with seasonings and bake at 350°F for 45 minutes.

WATER DINNER #1

Roasted Chicken Breast

1 roasting chicken

2 tbsp. fresh rosemary

10 cloves garlic

2 medium onions

2 tsp. olive oil

Preheat oven to 450°F. Place garlic and rosemary under the skin of breasts and drumsticks. Brush onions with olive oil and arrange around chicken. Insert meat thermometer into chicken prior to placing in the oven. Cook at 450°F for 30 minutes. Baste frequently. Remove chicken from oven when the meat thermometer registers at 180°F.

WATER DINNER #2

Lamb Kebobs

12 oz. lamb

2 tbsp. water

2 tbsp. Bragg's Amino Liquid

$^1/_2$ cup of pineapple juice

1 tsp. onion

1 garlic clove

$^1/_2$ cup pineapple cubes

$^1/_2$ cup red peppers/green peppers, cubed

Marinate lamb in water, Bragg's, pineapple juice, onion, and garlic. Place lamb and last two ingredients on skewers and grill until cooked through.

WATER DINNER #3

Grilled Veal Dinner

1 tsp. olive oil

1 pound veal scaloppini

$^1/_4$ tsp. salt

$^1/_4$ tsp. pepper

Brush oil over veal, and sprinkle with salt and pepper. Cook 2 minutes on each side or until done. Arrange veal on top of mashed sweet potatoes and butternut squash.

Mashed Sweet Potatoes and Butternut Squash

2 medium sweet potatoes

1 medium butternut squash, cut into halves

$1/2$ tsp. sea salt

$1/2$ tsp. pepper

$1/2$ tsp. cinnamon

$1/2$ tsp. nutmeg

$1/2$ tsp. allspice

$1/2$ tsp. ginger

1 tbsp. fresh lemon juice

2 tbsp. rice syrup

Preheat oven to 350°F. Put the butternut squash halves upside down on a cookie sheet. Place in oven with the sweet potatoes until both are soft, about 45 min., then let cool. Scoop out the insides of the squash and potatoes. Mash together with the remaining ingredients.

Five Simple
Ta'i Ch'i Exercises

T a'i ch'i can be thought of as a moving meditation because it's a form of physical exercise that promotes a deep, meditative relaxation in both the body and the mind. This is accomplished through various mind/body mechanisms that trigger the release of biochemicals into the body when the mind is relaxed. These chemicals, including an array of neuropeptides and immune enhancers, such as interferon, have a decidedly healing effect on the mind/body.

In simple terms, ta'i ch'i balances the body's life-force energy, or ch'i, which results in better health and well-being.

Ta'i ch'i promotes flexibility and strength, both physically and mentally. It's a gentle form of exercise that can be practiced by people of any age. Ta'i ch'i helps to rebuild both the spirit and the body and will impart a gratefulness to the mind and body while improving health in a variety of ways, including better breathing, better digestion, increased blood circulation, increased lung function, and lower blood pressure.

Ultimately, ta'i ch'i improves overall health by stimulating a strong flow of ch'i throughout the mind/body.

Should you become uncomfortable while practicing these positions, don't become alarmed. It is normal for you to feel some shaking or perhaps feel hot or cold. If you become nauseous or dizzy, you may find that you are hungry or tired. If this is the case, stop and drink some hot tea, or eat something light, and relax a while before continuing with the exercises. Do not expose yourself to cold or direct wind while doing these exercises as this may make you vulnerable to a cold or flu as a result of energetic weakness.

It is important that you don't try to breathe in any special way—your breath should be natural and effortless. During practice, you may keep your eyes open or closed, whichever way feels most comfortable for you.

I learned the following ta'i ch'i exercises from my dear friend, Master Tom Tam, whose guidance has enhanced my work and life.

EXERCISE 1. WU-CH'I—BEFORE THE BEGINNING

Stand with your feet shoulder width apart. Let your arms hang from your shoulders loosely, hands at your sides, with the palms facing back.

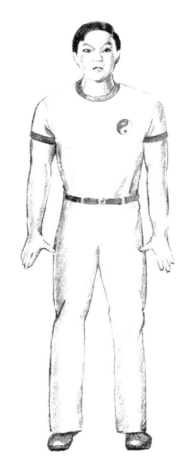

Your hands should be open and relaxed, not stretched or straightened tensely. Bend your knees slightly as if you were about to sit on a tall stool—the slight bend of your knees will cause your hips to tilt forward, straightening the inward curve in the small of your back. Keep your head erect, tilted slightly forward as though it were suspended on a string attached to its center. Touch the tip of your tongue to the palate where your teeth and gums meet. This connection between your tongue and palate completes an energy circuit that helps with the smooth flow of ch'i. Your weight should be evenly distributed between your toes and heels.

Your eyes can be either open or closed. Some people feel dizzy with their eyes closed. If this occurs, just open your eyes, and the sensation should pass within five to ten minutes. Breathe naturally through your nose. Relax your entire body and let the weight of it sink into the floor. You may visualize a waterfall flowing through it—the water enters through the top of your head, slowly washing the tension from every muscle and organ of your body as it flows down toward your toes. After the water soothes your feet, imagine it disappearing into the ground.

As you relax, your breathing will begin to calm and you will start to feel more centered and grounded. Initially, you may feel nothing, or perhaps a tingling or feeling of heat in your palms or elsewhere in your body. This is a normal reaction, the natural feeling of ch'i beginning to move in your body. When you feel ch'i, refrain from becoming overly excited or frightened, just let the feeling take its course.

This stance is called wu ch'i, or ma bu. Through the stillness of your body, you can feel the internal movement of ch'i. This state of being is called "outside silence and inside vibration." You can stand in this posture for five to ten minutes, or longer, if you enjoy the movement. Do not underestimate the value or importance of this stance just because there is no outward movement. Practicing it will bring mental and physical benefits of relaxation and renewed energy in a short period of time.

EXERCISE 2. THE BEGINNING OF TA'I CH'I

Begin by gently turning your hands palms up and raising them, slowly and softly, to shoulder height. Allow your shoulder joint to lift your upper arm, elbow, forearm, wrist, and hand. When your hands reach shoulder height, your palms should be facing upward toward the sky, as though holding ch'i from the universe.

Your arms will be extended and your elbows bent (not locked). Gauge the extension of your arms so that your shoulders, elbow, and wrists are comfortable. At their highest point, the wrists and elbows should be equidistant from the ground. Your arms should be slightly bent and your elbows lower than your wrists and shoulders. Allow gravity to pull your elbows down into a comfortable position. This movement should be gentle, slow, and soft. There should be no resistance in your arms and shoulders.

When resistance is low and your position is relaxed, bioelectricity moves more freely. It is not uncommon for people to experience shaking, tingling, or heat in their hands and body when doing this movement. It is the release of habitual tension and is a natural consequence of ch'i.

According to Chinese medical philosophy, there are six meridian pathways along each arm. Three originate in the torso and upper arm and run all the way to the tip of the fingers, and three originate at the tip of the fingers and run back to the torso and head. When ch'i moves, different meridians have different reactions.

When your arms are raised to shoulder height, turn your hands over softly, so that your palms are perpendicular with the ground. Gently lower your arms, tilting your hands slightly as your arms get closer to your waist. Use the same speed lowering your arms as you did raising them. When your hands are in the wu' position, begin the movement

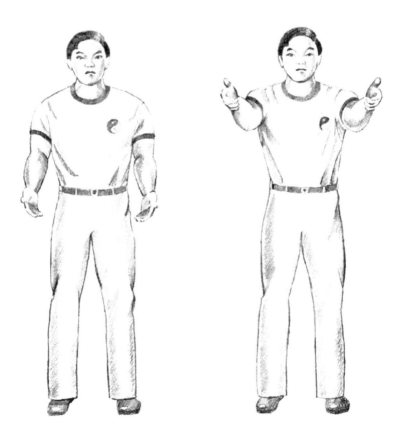

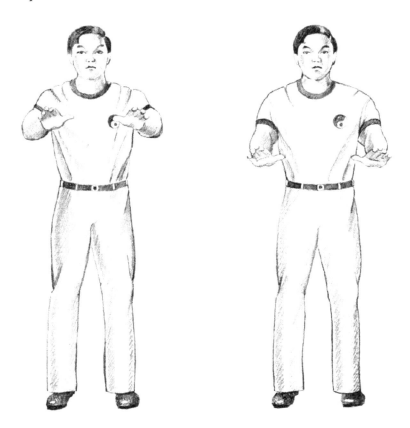

again. Raise and lower the hands six times, in multiple sets of six, as long as you remain comfortable doing so. If you begin to feel uncomfortable (nauseous or dizzy), return to the starting position and relax.

Now that you understand the mechanics of the exercises, think about their meaning. When the palms raise and face upward, you are gathering energy from the sky or heaven. This is yang energy. When your hands reach shoulder level and your palms turn down toward the ground, it's the end of yang energy and the start of gathering yin energy from the Earth. It's important that each time the yin movement is done, your hands return to the wu ch'i beginning posture.

Again, do not be alarmed if your body shakes or heats up. It is eliminating excessive tension in order to return to a balanced state. Move, shake, release the heat, the cold, the wind, the dampness, and after it's gone, you will feel much better.

EXERCISE 3. BRINGING THE CH'I DOWN TO THE DANTIEN

Raise your right hand up to the level of your head, with your palm perpendicular to the front of your body. Again, allow the shoulder joint to lift your upper arm, elbow, forearm, wrist, and hand, in that order. Turn your palm toward your body and lower it to your abdomen, keeping your hand six to eight inches from your body. This is where the dantien, the body's center of gravity and the *storage tank* for the body's internal ch'i energy, is located. It is approximately three inches below the navel and one to two inches below the surface of the skin. There are differing opinions concerning the precise location of the dantien, but everyone agrees that it is located in the abdominal area.

Now, raise your left hand slowly up to the level of your head, keeping your palm perpendicular to the front of your body. Remember that your shoulder lifts the rest of your arm. Turn your palm toward your body and lower it to the dantien. Continue to alternate hands until each hand has brought the energy to the dantien six times.

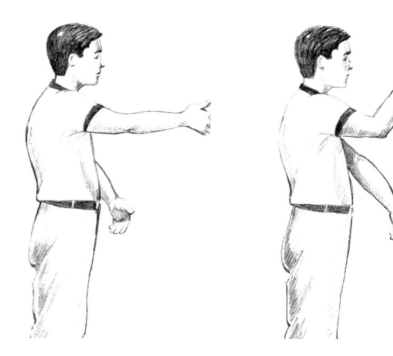

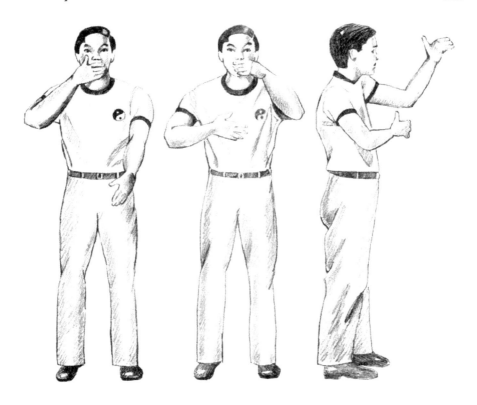

Many beginners have a difficult time coordinating the movement of two hands at the same time. If you find this routine difficult, you can try moving first one hand and then the other. Or you can try imagining that you are climbing a rope or a pole—while one hand is going up, the other hand is going down, and your two hands move in front of you in a circular motion.

EXERCISE 4. LEADING THE CH'I TO THE PALM

Raise your left arm to shoulder height with your palm facing the sky. Your wrist is no higher than your shoulder, and your elbow is slightly bent. Place the palm of your right hand two to four inches above your heart. Then, starting at your left shoulder, gently move your right hand down the length of your left arm. At the same time, your left elbow bends and lowers, pulling your left palm back. Keep a two- to four-inch distance between your right palm and your left arm as your right palm moves down your left arm.

Your left palm moves to the left side of your body, finishing the movement at your waist. Your palm still faces the sky. Your right palm extends forward, always at shoulder height. Your elbow is not locked when your

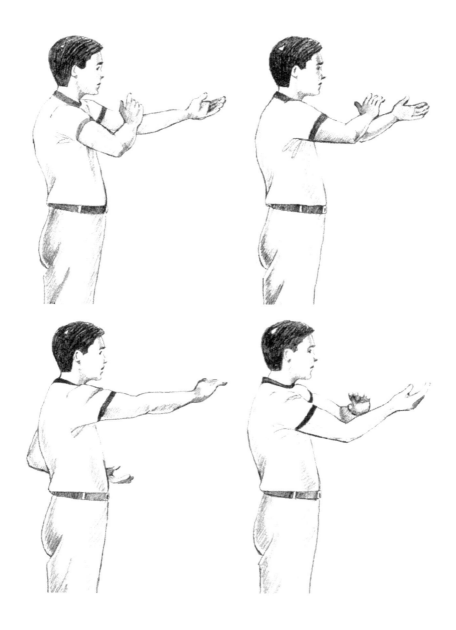

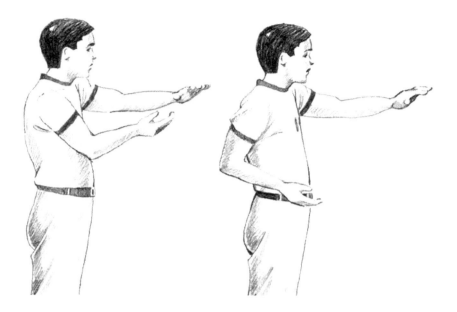

right arm is extended beyond the fingertips of your left hand. Your right arm extends, finishing the movement with your palm facing the earth, your wrist in line with, and no higher than, your right shoulder, with your elbows slightly bent.

Next, rotate the wrist of your right hand so that your palm faces the sky. Place your left palm two to four inches above your heart. Gently move your left hand toward your right shoulder and down the length of your right arm as your right elbow bends and lowers, pulling your palm back. Now, rotate the wrist of your left hand so your palm faces the sky.

This movement makes people feel calm and relaxed because the pericardium meridian in Chinese medicine helps to regulate emotional and psychological well-being. If you like, you can do this movement for five to fifteen minutes.

EXERCISE 5. HOLDING THE CH'I AT THE DANTIEN

Widen your stance to about one and a half times the width of your shoulders. Imagine sitting on a shorter stool. This will help you tilt your pelvis slightly forward so that your spine remains straight. Place both hands, right over left or left over right, on the dantien, located three inches below the navel. Some people feel more comfortable with their right hand closest to their body. Some like their left hand closest to their body. Everyone is different. You can experiment to see which side feels more natural. After you have made this com-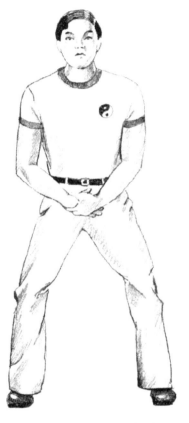parison, for future practice keep in mind which one felt more comfortable.

Once your hands are situated, breathe naturally six times, or for one to two minutes. If you feel good during this posture, you can remain in it as long as you like. If you stand too long, though, you may experience shaking or aching in the legs, so don't force yourself. Hold this position only as long as it feels comfortable. The top of your head and your tailbone should be in a straight line. Make sure your breath is natural and effortless.

Keeping your palms overlapped in the same position, lift them two to four inches away from the dantien. Rotate your palms six times around the dantien in a clockwise direction. Repeat the rotation six times in a counterclockwise direction. Continue rotating six times in a clockwise direction, then six times in a counterclockwise direction until you have completed three repetitions in each direction. Be sure to do the rotation slowly and gently.

The dantien stores ch'i and expands and contracts as your internal energy is gathered and released. You must try to keep the tank full, but never stagnant. This form, practiced regularly, will move the ch'i and keep clear the pathways through which the ch'i flows. Ch'i is healing energy. If ch'i is allowed to flow freely, good health results.

PART 3

The Contemporary West

13

The Contemporary West

If there is one bridge that is fast emerging as the most fundamental link between the ancient East and the contemporary West, it is food.

While the concept of food as therapy has long been disregarded by the contemporary West, it was one of the original eight sacred healing therapies of the ancient Chinese. Established some 6,000 years ago, food medicine is said to have been introduced by the great leader Shen Wung.

Today, through the growing science of nutrition, the West is *finally* embracing the healing qualities of food. With this, the ancient Chinese teachings have come full circle to flower anew in today's West. With more than 6,000 nutritional studies being conducted annually, people are at long last becoming aware of the profound impact that food plays in disease and healing.

Nutritional science first began to gain the respect of the West through evidence that linked dietary fats, most specifically cholesterol, with an increased risk for heart disease and high blood pressure. Since that time, nutritional science has more solidly established the therapeutic value of healthy foods in helping to reverse a host of degenerative diseases.

The public's desire for this knowledge is reflected in the immense amount of coverage the popular press gives these nutritional studies. Nutrients, such as vitamins, minerals, trace minerals, proteins, fats, carbohydrates, amino acids, essential fatty acids, and most recently, phytonutrients, are among the list of natural healing superstars. Almost daily, new studies reveal a different food's ability to enhance health, healing, longevity, peak performance, and youthfulness. Pick up any magazine or newspaper and see the headlines: "Anti-aging Breakthrough," "Sleep Better With Natural Remedies," or "Ease Allergies Without Drugs." Today, quite by surprise, the West has made food its new super medicine. By doing this, it has built a bridge from its Western scientific home base to the intuitive wisdom of the ancient East.

Today, the West is taking up where the first nutritionists left off so long ago, and at last there is an open flow of communication from both East and West. Today, the West is no longer a one-dimensional mechanistic information base. It is, at last, demonstrating a willingness to consider more options. Because of this, many futurists project that, in the coming years, alternative medicine, specifically nutrition, has the most profound potential for growth of any treatment area. This isn't surprising when you consider how much Westerners prize independence and self-control. These qualities are very much in keeping with the tenets of nutritional therapy, including responsibility for your own health, illness prevention, the cultivation of peak performance, and longevity. With far fewer—and often no—side effects, nutritional science holds the key to the future. What those of the ancient East knew instinctively, the people of the contemporary West have rediscovered through their intellect. And in the spirit of wholism, East and West will, by working together, usher health and natural healing into the future.

14

Basic Dietary Principles for Maximum Healing

IT ALL BEGINS WITH DIGESTION

Creating vibrant health begins with good digestion, yet Americans spend two billion dollars each year on antacids. And while taking alkalizers may relieve the discomfort of heartburn, it does *nothing* to aid digestion.

It's all well and good to eat healthy foods, but if your digestion is inadequate you will get little benefit from even the most nutritious diet, and poor digestion is one of the root causes of most degenerative illnesses.

What is considered digestion can be more accurately described as the seven stages of food transformation. These stages, which accomplish the transformation of foods into compounds the body can use, include:

1. Ingestion
2. Digestion
3. Absorption
4. Transportation
5. Respiration
6. Metabolism
7. Excretion

The digestive breakdown process is both mechanical (chewing, muscular contraction, and peristalsis) and chemical (digestive enzymes breaking the food down into usable substances). The transformation of food is accomplished in the gastrointestinal tract, which is twenty-five to thirty feet long and extends from the mouth to the anus.

The process begins with ingestion in the mouth, where chewing increases the surface area of a bite-sized piece of food, thus creating more access for digestive enzymes to do their work. Several glands produce mylase and pryalin, digestive enzymes designed to break down carbohydrates. It is interesting to note that carbohydrates are the first food group to begin to be digested, which suggests that the quick energy they provide helps fuel the long and laborious process referred to simply as digestion.

From the mouth, the partially digested food travels through the esophagus to the stomach by the action of gravity and peristalsis, an involuntary wavelike muscular motion. In the stomach, food mixes with hydrochloric acid and pepsin, which begins the process of breaking down fats and proteins.

A valvelike structure called the cardiac sphincter controls the entrance of food into the stomach and also prevents hydrochloric acid from splashing back up into the esophagus. When there is trouble in this area, it can often feel as though the pain is coming from the heart. Furthermore, indigestion of this type can initiate heart arrhythmias and hiatal hernias.

From the stomach, food enters the small intestine, which is approximately twenty feet long and has three major sections. It is the work of the small intestine to finish digesting all three food groups: fats, carbohydrates, and proteins. Although the liver, gallbladder, and pancreas are not part of the gastrointestinal tract, they each contribute to digestion by secreting substances into the small intestine that are essential to the process. It is in the small intestine that nutrients are absorbed from the gastrointestinal tract into the blood and the lymph systems, which distribute them throughout the body. The liver produces bile for fat emulsification, while the gallbladder stores bile from the liver and is also capable of secreting it into the small intestine as needed. The pancreas secretes a variety of enzymes that are essential for the digestion of fats, carbohydrates, and proteins.

From the small intestine, the non-digestible remnants, or ash, of the food we eat pass into the large intestine, or colon. The solid wastes formed here contain bacteria, cholesterol, dead cells, food residue, fungi, unabsorbed minerals, and yeast. No digestion occurs here. This waste then collects in the rectum and passes from the body via the anal canal.

STRESS AND PH

The mind/body moves and changes through time, in sync with a number of cyclical rhythms triggered by light, temperatures, and certain internal phenomena. Among them are a seven-day biorhythmic cycle and a twenty-eight-day cycle. There's also a twenty-four hour metabolic cycle, during which certain hours are favored for particular body functions. For instance, digestion is best accomplished by the body between the hours of 7 a.m. and 3 p.m., while tissue building takes place between 3 p.m. and 11 p.m. The third cycle, which occurs between the hours of 11 p.m. and 7 a.m., is when the body naturally cleanses cellular wastes.

One of the most important cycles in terms of health is the pH (potential hydrogen) cycle, which measures the acid-alkaline chemical balance in the body. While it is normal for the body's pH to fluctuate as part of a daily pH cycle, acid-alkaline balance must remain within a narrow range in order to sustain life. Within this narrow range, there is an optimum balance point that indicates a healthy state. The body's pH is measured in all the body fluids. Blood pH is the principle guiding indicator. Blood pH should range from between 7.2–7.4. If yours is below 7.2, you are far too acid and most likely very ill, and if it is above 7.4 you are far too alkaline and also likely to be very ill. A balanced pH indicates a healing state, while excesses in either extreme indicate an environment ripe for disease.

The easiest vehicle for monitoring pH is urine. The scale for urine pH is different from that of blood, but it corresponds with blood's. Urine pH ranges from 5.0–7.0, with the healthy balance point between 6.4–6.8. Thus, a urinary pH of 6.4–6.8 tells you that your blood pH is exactly balanced between 7.3 and 7.4.

Urinary pH that is consistently *well below* 6.4 indicates a very acidic, fiery condition in the body. This reflects a hyper-stress environment that predisposes a person toward such illnesses as diabetes, fibromyalgia, lupus, rheumatoid arthritis, and a variety of cancers. On the other hand, a urinary pH consistently *well above* 6.8 indicates a hyper-alkaline environment that usually reflects a broken-down, deficient condition caused by extreme stress over along period of time. This predisposes a person to diarrhea, heart disease, immune deficiency, indigestion, and melancholia.

Most people these days are affected by overly acidic conditions. Stress causes the body to produce stress hormones and other acids that contribute to this, so controlling stress is key to bringing an acidic pH into balance. Overindulging in processed, high-starch, dead carbohydrates and fatty proteins creates acidic conditions, and eating at least two large servings of cholorophyll-rich, leafy, green vegetables each day will help a hyper-acid pH.

To test your urinary pH, I recommend using the .067 pHydrion paper strips that measure urine pH from 5.5–8.0. They are available in health food stores and some pharmacies, and they are made by Micro Essential Laboratory, Inc. The company's website is microessentiallab.com. Test your first urine of the day by letting it run across a several inch strip of the pHydrion paper, then immediately compare its color to the chart on the container.

To regulate an overly *acid* pH, you can try the following, depending on your bio-individuality and the state of your constitution:

- Aerobic exercise

- Chlorophyll capsules, two, twice a day

- Cold baths and showers

- Deep breathing

- Epsom salt baths

- Fresh vegetable juice

- Herbal teas, especially alfalfa

- Lemon juice and water

- Raw salads

- Ta'i ch'i

- Yoga exercise

To regulate an overly *alkaline* pH, you can try the following, depending on your bio-individuality and the state of your constitution:

- Brisk walks

- Herbal teas, especially spearmint

- Hot baths and showers

- Multi-digestive enzymes

- Papain-bromelain enzymes

- Raw acid foods, including grapefruit, papaya, and pineapple

Since stress plays such a large role in creating disease and blocking health, it's important to understand the dynamics of the stress response. Many people use the words stress and stressed-out frequently, but few know what they actually mean.

FIGHT OR FLIGHT STRESS RESPONSE— GENERAL ADAPTATION SYNDROME

Fight or flight, the stress response, evolved to help ancient human beings adapt to the world they lived in. Primitive cave dwellers who frequently encountered a number of life-and-death situations needed to be able to respond fast and powerfully to sudden events. The stress response gave them the energy they needed to accomplish feats they would have been unable to accomplish under normal circumstances.

Although today there's no saber-toothed tiger around to outsmart or any mastodon to run from, people are equipped with the same response system as their primitive ancestors.

Interestingly, it doesn't matter what the stressful situation actually is that shifts people into the fight or flight mode. What matters is how they perceive or interpret the situation. Whatever they see as threatening, what they become anxious about, and what makes them angry or impatient, all turn on the stress response. Instantaneously, such perceptions activate chemical messages that travel from the brain's hypothalamus, pineal gland, amygdala and the sensory cortex, and on throughout the body.

These chemical messages communicate an entirely different set of instructions than the ones used for healthy, normal living (homeostasis). In this stress condition, the body's priority is to manufacture as much energy as it can, as fast as it can. All other functions not crucial to producing immediate energy in response to the perceived emergency are suspended.

The second the hypothalamus (the stress sensor) perceives the initial stress, the pituitary gland activates the adrenal glands to produce a number of stress hormones that begin the first of three stages of redirecting physiological activities.

Stage 1. In the first (acute) stage of alarm reaction, the adrenal hormones send the message to the body to increase the heart rate to prepare the body machine for increased inertia. Next, the peripheral blood vessels in the hands, feet, and skin are constricted so the internal vital organs can receive more blood. Then the spleen contracts, and blood clotting increases to offset any potential for excessive bleeding. The liver's glycogen stores are released in order to increase the energy supply, and sweat production is increased to lower the rising body temperature. Breathing steps up, and the respiratory passageways expand to facilitate oxygen intake, which, in turn, allows the body to eliminate the excess carbon dioxide from catabolism (tissue breakdown for energy). Finally, saliva and enzyme releases are decreased as digestion is not necessary.

Stage 2. Then, if stress persists, the second resistance-response stage (chronic stress) engages. Through the cholinergic response, large stores of hydrochloric acid are released that are designed to burn food quickly so the body can fight, or flee, more efficiently. This causes blood pH to become very acidic, which is conducive to the energy-burning function that becomes the body's top priority during the stress response.

Having burned through its food sources, the body then begins to withdraw protein from the thymus and lymph glands to break *it* down for use as immediate energy. Quite a bit of calcium is lost through this process, since almost 50 percent of the body's calcium is bonded with proteins, which act as the body's Public Works Department, constantly fixing and repairing the body. During the stress response, all normal repair and maintenance work is suspended, as the body diverts all proteins for use as energy (this withdrawal of protein from these critical glands is a powerfully destructive process). Additionally, excess sugars store in the liver as starch or glycogen, ready to be instantly reconverted to energy on demand.

As part of this process, blood pressure rises to facilitate the flow of energy to vital organs. Because the normal work of proteins is halted, the body withdraws minerals from the bones to use for repair work. More calcium, so crucial to strong bones, is lost in this way, as are other minerals, including magnesium, essential for calming nerves. Again, the body is almost cannibalizing itself to mobilize all the energy it can to respond to the stress situation. Fat is also called upon to be used as quick energy, and sodium is retained in order to help the body hold on to its water reserves and prevent dehydration.

The fight-or-flight response was designed to be used in emergency situations lasting very short periods of time. It is essential that it be turned off as soon as possible to allow the body to return to its normal health-maintaining activities.

The stress response wasn't meant to go on for long periods of time, so when the stress response becomes chronic, you end up depleting all the excess reserves in your organs. You can no longer pull protein from exhausted glands because there is none left, nor can you take calcium from broken-down bone tissue. In this stage, the body has shifted to another strategy to get the immediate energy it needs, namely diverting every bit of food for use as immediate energy. Normally, a portion of food is used immediately, while the rest goes into a number of building and storing processes. Among these are the maintenance of the immune system, routine repair work, and the routine storage of energy for future use. During this stage of the stress response, however, none of these normal, important activities can take place because the body, having depleted all its reserves, has nowhere to turn for energy except the food that it eats.

Stage 3. Once Stage 2 becomes chronic, the body becomes completely exhausted and passes into a Stage 3 state of acute stress response. At this point, the mind/body is extremely depleted and deficient. This is a state of extreme exhaustion that can sometimes lead to death.

STRESS DIGESTION

As I've emphasized, stress has a powerfully damaging effect on the mind/body, which includes digestion. When experts talk about digestion, or writers describe it in textbooks, they refer to digestion in an ideal person who lives a peaceful life and has a calm mind/body. Unfortunately, this applies to few Americans today.

The human body was designed to live in a calm, sympathetic-dominant state of being 90 percent of the time, with the capacity to shift into the fight-or-flight stress response mode approximately 10 percent of the time, as needed. Unfortunately, today it is just the opposite, with the vast majority of people spending 90 percent of their time in a stressed, fight-or-flight mode, and only 10 percent of their time feeling relaxed and easy.

Because of this, I believe that today there are two kinds of digestion. One is the healthy digestion of a mostly stress-free person, and the other is the digestion of the acutely stressed, which I refer to as *stress digestion*. Eating a wonderful diet will do little for you if you are in a acute state of stress.

Chronic Stage 2 stress causes the body to overproduce hydrochloric acid to burn through food very quickly in order to sustain the emergency stress mode. The chronic overproduction of hydrochloric acid, however, depletes these digestive juices, leaving inadequate stores for later use. Yet without hydrochloric acid, the body cannot begin to digest proteins, fats, calciums, and a number of other substances, so digestion is immeasurably impaired. Consequently, partially digested proteins end up putrefying in the large intestines, while partially digested carbohydrates ferment. In theory, foods such as broccoli have the potential to be powerfully medicinal, but any food that stays in the body longer than the normal transit period of 28–36 hours becomes a pathogen.

Impaired digestion leads the way to numerous degenerative diseases, but this is only the half of it. Not only does chronic stress suppress the production of the digestive aid hydrochloric acid, stress also produces enormous neuroendocrine imbalances throughout the body that impact the digestive process by affecting the blood pressure as well as the gall-bladder, heart, intestines, liver, and pancreas.

Fight or flight is geared toward supplying the mind/body with extra energy. It accomplishes much of this through the combined action of the adrenal hormones, which redirect the action of most of the body's systems from all non-essential functions to survival. In doing so, these hormones also dilate blood vessels, raise blood pressure, and stimulate cardiac function, increasing the rate and force of the heart's contractions. In addition, they activate enzymes that promote glucose formation in the liver, while inhibiting the pancreatic production of insulin. Decreased insulin prevents glucose from being used by the tissue and increases its availability to the central nervous system. The adrenal hormones also mobilize fats for use in the fight and inhibit the breakdown of cholesterol.

Chronic adrenaline release raises blood-glucose levels, increasing the risk of adult-onset diabetes and hypoglycemia. It also speeds respiratory and metabolic rates, which increases the risk of thyroid and parathyroid problems. Additionally, chronic adrenaline release constricts the blood vessels in the intestine, further hampering protein digestion and assimilation, while dilating blood vessels in the muscles, which raises the risk of musculoskeletal debilitation. The depletion of adrenaline due to chronic stress also destroys adrenaline's ability to function as a crucial anti-inflammatory for neutralizing allergic and inflammatory reactions.

Through the combined working of all aspects of this stress response, a wide array of enzymes and hormones responsible for regulating normal processes are suppressed, including digestive-enzyme production, sex-hormone production, and the production and circulation of lymphocytes, white blood cells, and other components of the immune system. Additionally, stress adversely affects bone density, brain function, the cardiovascular system, genetic integrity, and wound repair.

BALANCING WILLIAM'S THYROID TO FIX HIS WEIGHT PROBLEM

William came to me when he was in his early thirties. He was 6'1" and had weighed only 138 pounds for his entire adult life. No matter what he tried, everything from protein powders to high-fat, high-carbohydrate foods, he couldn't gain any weight. A while after I met William, he bought his first house and then almost immediately lost his job. Suddenly, he was thrown into an acute state of stress. After having a secure source of money, he had no income for the first time in his life and was terribly worried that he wouldn't be able to make his house payments.

In a very short time, William shot up to 220 pounds. This incredible weight gain was the result of a change in the activity of his thyroid. Normally responsible for controlling fatty metabolism, William's thyroid had previously been *overactive*. After the onset of his stress, however, his routine thyroid activity was diverted from its normal metabolic functioning to supporting the needs of the stress response. Thus, his thyroid became *underactive* as a calorie burning mechanism and he gained nearly 80 pounds.

Once I balanced his thyroid metabolism, his weight stabilized at the right level for him and it has remained stable ever since. Today, William is strong, fit, and, energetic.

The preceding effects of the stress response reflect just a smattering of the functions that become disrupted and neglected during the fight-or-flight response. What is essential to understand is that this response is designed to last *short* periods of time to allow the body to respond to an acute, emergency situation. It is essential to wellness that this potentially destructive response mode be turned off as soon as possible. Clearly, stress is not just something that makes us a little tired. It is a very real, potentially destructive force. Unfortunately, life today and the often unconscious decision to go fast, get more, and generally "keep up with the Joneses" has caused many to live in a near-constant state of fight or flight. It is up to every person to become more committed to peace of mind and body. In order to respond to the healing qualities of food, people need to shift out of stress digestion into normal, healthy, stress-free digestion capable of delivering the essential nutrients on which minds and bodies depend.

BIO-INDIVIDUALITY

No Diet Is Right for Everyone All the Time

It is important to understand that because each individual has specific and unique nutritional needs, no single diet is right for everyone. Additionally, each person is subject to constantly changing conditions, and what might be good for you during one period might not be so good for you during another.

The chapters on the five constitutional types introduced you to the concept of individual constitutional types as used by various cultures, including the ancient Chinese. These systems, used to differentiate among people's unique constitutions, helped individuals and healers to better understand the energetic nature of a person and his or her corresponding tendencies, strengths, and weaknesses. Knowing if you are high strung and tend toward excitability, or whether you are more likely to withdraw, feel cold, and have little appetite, helps tailor your diet to the foods that are best for your individual constitution.

This bio-individuality accounts for the fact that so many widely differing, often contrary, diet systems are popular today; some are good for some people, and some are good for others. Popular diets that emphasize protein, other diets that stress carbohydrates, and still others that recommend only raw foods, are all valid and valuable for some types and not for others. It is essential, then, that each person find a way to tailor the following basic dietary guidelines to their particular constitutions and intolerances (allergic reactions). I use the five constitutional types that are presented earlier in the book, as well as AK (applied kinesiology) testing, a system that reads the body's subtle electrical muscular responses, to determine if a particular food is tolerable for a person at a particular time. There are a number of other methods to determine your individual nutritional approach and what foods are best for you, including cytotoxic or scratch testing, Elisa testing, food rotation, and vega testing (a mechanical biofeedback method).

If you are working with the five constitutional types, you may want to modify the basic diet by using more foods from the food flavor group that corresponds with your type.

For example, if you are a fire type in a high-energy mode, you will want to use more bitter vegetables (good for reducing inflammatory conditions) rather than a full range of vegetables. If, on the other hand, you are a water type in an exhausted state, you may need to increase your intake of protein foods. There is always room to adjust the basic dietary guidelines to adapt better to the changing needs in your life.

In the basic program that follows, I present several aspects of the basic dietary guidelines that I believe to be fundamental starting points for a healthy diet. These guidelines are intended for use when you're feeling fine. When and if you are ill or experiencing an acute health crisis, I would recommend a more strictly curative diet. I will explain further as we go on.

THE BASIC PROGRAM OF DIETARY GUIDELINES

To begin with, I categorize all foods into one of three major groups.

- The first group, *toxic foods,* includes all processed sugary and snack-style junk foods, plus highly carcinogenic cured deli meats and bacon. This toxic food group also includes all intolerable, allergenic foods. It is important to realize that each person has different food intolerances and allergies unique to them. Often you may think you don't have any allergies if you don't have typical allergic reactions, but food intolerances and allergies can have less obvious, but equally debilitating, effects. Food intolerances can be the cause of backaches, headaches, indigestion, and a wide array of other health problems.

- The second group, *neutral foods,* are those which are not directly disease-producing, but which have no healing potential, such as white pasta and white rice.

- The third group, *therapeutic foods,* includes a wide range of fruits and vegetables, whole grains, legumes, and certain lean protein sources you are not allergic to.

As a general guideline, I recommend that people strive to consume a ratio of at least 70 percent therapeutic foods, and no more than 15 percent each of the neutral and toxic groups. I call this my 85 percent rule, which suggests that you try to eat wholesome (neutral or therapeutic) foods 85 percent of the time.

I also break foods down into three categories in terms of individual digestion.

- The first group I call *tolerance foods,* which are those foods that you can eat on a daily basis and digest well.

- The second category are *swing foods,* those foods that you can digest only on an occasional basis. Eating too much of a swing food often pushes it into the intolerance category, while abstaining from it for a period may allow you to regain your tolerance.

- The third category, *intolerance foods,* are those that act as allergens. No matter how little you eat of an intolerance food, you cannot digest it.

The average person's diet is about 65 percent tolerance foods, 25 percent swing foods, and 10 percent intolerance foods.

Having divided foods into these three categories, I then make my dietary recommendations according to food groups. I recommend that 65 percent of your daily calorie intake be comprised of vegetables, fruits, and whole, unrefined grains and grain products (brown rice, millet, oats, quinoa, rye). Fats should comprise 20–25 percent of your intake, the majority of which should be mono- and polyunsaturated oils: safflower, sesame, sunflower, and vegetable. Finally, 12–15 percent of your intake should consist of low-fat animal and vegetable proteins. (Keep in mind that these percentages are general guidelines. Each person should be screened to determine her or his individual needs.) I also recommend eating fruits more frequently when they are in season—between May and November in temperate climates.

Food preparation should also be in balance with the seasons so that cold, raw foods are served more in the late spring and summer, while warm, cooked foods are preferred in the fall and winter. Cooking methods and the use of raw versus cooked foods can also be determined by the person's constitutional type and his or her needs at a particular time. In general, however, I recommend cooked foods over raw, as proper cooking destroys pathogens while increasing many nutrient yields and decreasing phlegm production in the body. Cooking methods—baking, boiling, braising, broiling, poaching, and sautéing—should be varied to produce a varied abundance of nutrients.

Cleaning Out the Kitchen Cabinets

The following items tend to fall into the toxic and intolerant food category and I recommend avoiding them whenever possible:

- All sugar. Corn sweeteners, dextrose, glucose, honey, maltose, maple syrup, molasses, raisin syrup, sucrose, turbinado sugar, and anything made from them;

- Any and all fried foods, white flour products, including white flour pasta, and other processed carbohydrates, such as buns, crackers, doughnuts, pizza, rolls, sweet rolls, white rice, and even chewing gum (sugar-free or otherwise);

- Soft drinks, (sugar-free or otherwise); cake, cookies; ice cream; sweetened juices;

- Condiments, such as gravies, jams, jellies, ketchup, mayonnaise, and relish;

- Excessively fatty foods, such as chowders, cream soups, and sour cream;

- Alcohol and caffeinated drinks of any kind;

- Additionally, I recommend reducing corn, dairy, and wheat because of their high concentration of allergens;

- Yeasted breads and baked goods should be replaced with yeast-free, sourdough products;

- Vinegars should be replaced with sulfite-free lemon and lime juices;

- Since fermented foods can escalate immuno-suppressive yeast in the body, I believe that all fermented soy-type sauces should be replaced with Bragg's Amino Liquid—this protein concentrate, derived from healthy soybeans, contains sixteen amino acids in naturally occurring amounts and is very similar in taste and function to soy sauce, but healthier for you;

- Peanuts contain the potentially toxic aflatoxin mold, while almonds are aflatoxin-free, so peanuts and peanut butters should be replaced by almonds and almond butters.

Food Combining

Over the years, there have been many studies substantiating the value of eating certain food groups *with* certain food groups and not with others. Most notable is the work of Dr. Herbert M. Shelton, who compiled extensive research on the topic from 1928–1981.[1]

Dr. Shelton's research was first noted in 1924 in the *Journal of American Medicine* by Dr. Philip Norman, who cited the effectiveness of proper food combining. My professional experience has led me to concur with this theory. I continually see the remarkable healing power of proper food combining, especially for those whose problems are traceable to digestive or metabolic difficulties.

Properly combined foods digest efficiently, whereas improperly combined foods may upset healthy digestion and nutrient assimilation. This is because different enzymes are required to break down various foods, and they can interfere with each other, causing nitrogen, methane, and hydrogen gases to ferment in the intestine.

The general rules of food combining are:

- Eat only one protein per meal

- Do not combine proteins with starches

- Do not combine fruits with any other foods

- Combine only fruits from within the same fruit group: acid, sub-acid, or sweet (*see* chart)

- Proteins combine well with low-starch vegetables (*see* chart)

- Low-starch vegetables combine well with starch vegetables

- Chew all food well

- Do not drink beverages during meals

- Drink beverages before meals or two hours afterwards

Figure 14.1. Food Combining Chart (on the following page) encapsulates the fundamentals of proper food combining.

THE ASSAULT ON FOOD PURITY—
PESTICIDES, TOXINS, GENETICALLY MODIFIED FOODS

Many in the West don't believe something unless they can see it, measure it, or test it. Consequently, the idea develops that if you can't see something, it can't hurt you. Sadly, there are many compounds in foods you can't see or taste that can have unhealthy effects on you.

You not only need to make the right choices concerning the foods you eat, but you also need to consider the quality of the foods themselves. If you know what farmers, producers, and manufacturers are doing to your food, you can make healthier choices at the marketplace, thus registering your preferences and requirements with every dollar you spend. And, should you feel so inclined, you can also be more vocal and active in the struggle to reclaim purer growing conditions for the food supply and fight any additional legislation that seeks to lower standards that are meant to safeguard the quality of foods.

Until the mid-1940s, American farmers used natural means to return vital nutrients to the soil, a practice that ensured nutritious food. After

FIGURE 14.1 FOOD COMBINING CHART

PROTEINS
(1 per meal)
beans, dairy, eggs,
fish, nuts, legumes,
meat, poultry, soy

Low Starch
VEGETABLES
celery, garlic, okra, onions,
peppers, summer squash,
asparagus, broccoli,
leafy greens

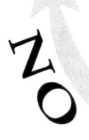 **YES**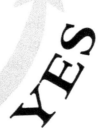

NO **YES**

High Starch **VEGETABLES**
beets, carrots, corn, parsnips, peas, potatoes, pumpkin, yams

High Starch **GRAINS**
breads, cereals, crackers, pastas, rice

Acid **FRUITS**	Sub Acid **FRUITS**	Sweet **FRUITS**
citrus, pineapple, kiwi, strawberry, tomato	apple, apricot, berries, cherries, grapes, melons, nectarine, pear, oranges, peach, papaya, plum	bananas, currants, dates, figs, raisins

All fruits taken alone and combined only with their groupings

the Second World War, however, things changed. Surplus chemicals used in the war, including nitrates and phosphates, found a homefront use as low-cost, high-yield chemical fertilizers. By the early 1960s, the American farm industry had totally converted to the synthetic fertilizers of today, depleting crops of vital nutrients.

Taking up where the farmer leaves off, manufacturers artificially supplement, can, dry, ferment, freeze, irradiate, pickle, preserve, salt, smoke, and sugar food. Even more damaging than these processes are the arsenal of chemicals added to food, including acidifiers, alkalizers, anti-foaming agents, bleaches, buffers, caking agents, deodorant, drying agents, dyes, emulsifiers, flavor enhancers, fortifiers, gases, hydrogenators, hydrolizers, preservatives, and sprays.

Unbelievably, this is not the end of the story. The most damaging practices involve pesticides and fungicides. Among the most dangerous are those with chlorinated hydrocarbon chains, including aldrin, DDT, endrin, and toxaphene. These chemicals don't break down, but rather continually recycle through food chains . . . and human bodies. Although DDT was banned by Congress in 1972, it continues to show up in dangerously high levels in certain seafoods.

Many pesticides still in use today are sprayed regularly on virtually every fruit and vegetable you see at the marketplace. Independent studies consistently find a horrifying number of chemical residues in these foods.

RECIPE TO COUNTERACT TOXINS

I recommend spritzing produce with two solutions.
First, use a mixture of 1 teaspoon cider vinegar in 10 ounces of water.
Follow this with a mixture of 1 teaspoon of baking soda in 10 ounces of water.
Use a final water rinse.
There are also rinses available at most natural foods stores.

Ideally, the government should assure the safety of the food supply, but the issue becomes tainted by greed, politics, confused priorities, and special interests. To make things worse, long-term human safety and safe exposure levels are unknown, yet it is the job of the Environmental Protection Agency (EPA) to determine the tolerance levels that are allowed for pesticide residues in foods. And it is the responsibility of the Food and Drug Administration and the Department of Agriculture to enforce these levels. The problem is that many scientists and researchers are constrained by politics, which leads to disagreement over what constitutes safe levels of these potentially dangerous toxins.

According to a study published by the National Institutes of Health, children aged 2–5 who ate non-organic produce had six times the level of pesticides in their urine compared to those who ate organic produce. The EPA states that children under two are ten times as likely to develop cancer as adults when exposed to certain gene-changing chemicals, while children ages 2–15 are three times as likely. The average child is exposed to 4–10 pesticides every day. For apples alone, after washing the average inorganic apple contains 4–5 pesticides.

In 1993, The National Academy of Sciences (NAS) found that the legal tolerance levels of exposure to pesticides for particular foods is for adults and *does not* guarantee the safety of children.

A late 1980s classic report by The Natural Resources Defense Council (NRDC) concluded that nearly three million American children are exposed to higher levels of neurotoxic pesticides than the EPA considers acceptable. Since tolerance levels are set with adults in mind, and children's bodies have consistently demonstrated dramatically different tolerances and reaction responses, the NRDC concluded that 5,500–6,200 preschoolers may eventually develop cancer as a result of childhood exposure to pesticides. Despite the fact that the NAS found the entire EPA regulatory system lacking and inadequate, not one of their recommendations have been adopted by the EPA, nor has Congress forced the EPA to do so.

Today, new processes that take the denaturalization of foods even further are being developed and introduced. Bovine growth hormone is now fed to dairy cows to make milk production higher. Frequently, this causes the animals to develop infected mammary glands requiring antibiotics that remain in the milk you drink. Genetic alterations are also in the works so that a tomato could possibly have animal genes in its flesh. Tragically, the law does not require the labeling of these products, so the only way you can be sure the dairy you are getting is free of synthetic hormones, or the tomato is purely vegetarian, is to buy organic, non-GMO products.

Genetically Modified Food—GMOs (Genetically Modified Organisms)

A GMO is an organism that has been genetically altered by genetic engineers who combine DNA molecules from different sources to create an entirely new set of genes. They then transfer the altered DNA into an organism in order to alter its properties. For example, thanks to genetic engineering, genes from a deepwater fish species are now being inserted into strawberries. This is because the fish has developed genes to protect it from the cold water temperatures, and by inserting these coldwater genes from the fish into the strawberry, their idea is to protect the strawberry from freeze damage.

This type of genetic modification is called *transgenic,* meaning that DNA was inserted from one species (in this case, animal) into another (in this case, fruit). Those organisms that have had DNA inserted from their own species, not another one, are called *cisgenic.*

Currently, there are more than 70 million acres of genetically modified crops in the world. More than 80 percent of those crops are modified to survive unlimited applications of herbicides. And there are even *herbicide crops* being engineered to produce their own pesticides genetically from within. There are also *terminator crops* being planted to produce sterile seeds, thus forcing farmers to purchase new seeds each year.

Corporate giant Monsanto currently owns 91 percent of the world's GMO market. Monsanto and other proponents argue that the technology will produce greater crop yields and will reduce the demand for water, fertilizer, and pesticides, making GMOs a plus for developing countries. Those against GMO technology are concerned, justifiably, that there is a great danger of drifting and the unintentional transfer of

GMO to non-GMO crops, which could ultimately reduce genetic diversity and all but eliminate wild crops and heirloom seeds.

GMOs pose a grave danger to anyone contending with serious food allergies and intolerances. I have worked with many thousands of chemically sensitive and allergy-prone men and women over the years who absolutely have to know exactly what they are eating at all times. This growing population that I continue to see reflects a world of diminished nutrient intake, increasing chronic stress, and systemic immunosuppression that the present healthcare system hasn't a clue how to prevent or treat.

The expansion of GMOs will have life-threatening consequences. For example, it's potentially deadly if someone who is severely, and perhaps anaphalactically, allergic to peanuts buys and eats an entirely different, apparently safe, food that, unbeknownst to them, has been genetically altered with peanut genes.

Many millions of people experience constipation, hay fever, insomnia, and migraine headaches due to food intolerances. It's bad enough that most of America is without a healthcare system to help them solve such problems. Now, even if they are fortunate enough to find effective healthcare for their conditions, they may never again know exactly what they're really eating.

Appallingly, there are currently no GMO labeling laws in North America.

Food allergies are on the rise globally. Since Great Britain began importing North American GMO soy, their incidences of food allergies have increased more than 50 percent. This irresponsible science has been confronted head-on by author Jeffrey Smith. In his groundbreaking book, *Seeds of Deception,* Smith puts a spotlight on the industry manipulation and political collusion behind GMO science.[2]

Smith reveals a history of scientific bribery, harassment of government officials, manipulated studies, and FDA information withheld from Congress. He explains how industry giant Monsanto is in a race to genetically modify the world's food supply. Apparently, they are well on their way. According to the Center for Food Safety, 45 percent of all U.S. corn is now GMO, as well as 85 percent of all U.S. soybeans, 72 percent of all cotton, and 75 percent of all processed foods. For a non-GMO shopping list, check out the website: seedsofdeception.com. (*See also* Resources in back)

And it doesn't end with food. America's drinking water is almost exclusively fluoridated. Although continually reassured by science that fluoridation prevents tooth decay and in no way jeopardizes anyone's well-being, there is mounting evidence to the contrary that *fluoride is toxic.*

The largest American study, involving more than 39,000 school children, concluded that fluoridation does *not,* in fact, reduce tooth decay in permanent teeth. Similar studies have taken place in New Zealand and Canada with similar results. Despite this, fluoride continues to appear in a number of products aside from the water supply, and is, in effect, in *all* drinks and cooked foods.

Fluoride has been readily documented as a toxic compound that many worldwide studies have linked to arthritis, cancer, collagen breakdown, genetic birth defects, osteoporosis, and skeletal fluorosis. A 1984 study published by Williams and Williams stated unequivocally that fluoride was more poisonous than lead and just slightly less toxic than arsenic.

In his book *Fit for Life II*, bestselling author Harvey Diamond reports that Dr. Dean Burke, former chief biochemist at the National Cancer Institute, stated on June 18, 1985, at an EPA meeting that "more than 50,000 Americans a year are dying of cancer caused by fluoridated drinking water."

In order to make the best choices for your family and friends, it is important to be aware of how the food and water supply is being adulterated. There is an alternative to this spreading problem because organically grown foods are now much more widely available everywhere in conventional supermarkets and natural food stores. Nearly every town and city has farmer's markets that offer organic foods and foods grown with fewer dangerous compounds.

Just as it is desirable to seek balance in all things, it is important to balance the response to this problem. I suggest you do your best to get the purest foods you can, while learning about the issues.

Fighting Cancer and Heart Disease with Food

The Top Twenty-Five Phytonutrient-Rich Super Foods

THE HEALING POWER OF FOODS

The vitamins and minerals in our foods have long been known to be capable of preventing a variety of diseases.

Today, the most exciting research substantiating the powerful healing properties of food involves a category of therapeutic compounds in fruits and vegetables called *phytonutrients*. These compounds, used by plants to protect themselves against various environmental stresses, have been found to have strong druglike powers to both reverse disease and prevent it. To date, nine families of phytonutrients, each of which contain hundreds of different compounds, have been identified.

Every fruit and every vegetable contains a variety of phytonutrients that act synergistically to most beneficially deliver the therapeutic compounds they contain. Whole foods are engineered by Nature to contain all the co-compounds necessary for the body to best utilize a particular food's beneficial formulas.

THE ANTIOXIDANT PROPERTIES OF PHYTONUTRIENTS

Among the phytonutrient's most valuable properties is its ability to act as an antioxidant, which are substances that counteract free-radical damage.

Free radicals are molecules that are missing an electron due to pollution, stress, or a variety of other natural and unnatural conditions. Because free radicals need an electron, they attack healthy cells and steal *theirs,* thus damaging the healthy cells. To make matters worse, this theft turns the newly attacked cells into unpaired, electron-lacking free radicals as well, creating a chain reaction that can cause cancer, heart disease, and other untold damage. In their quest to quench their thirst for an electron, free radicals attack *all* cells, including those in your genes.

Genes, made of DNA, are responsible for instructing cells how to behave. When DNA is strong and healthy, you are strong and healthy. However, DNA is comprised of long strands of molecules that are easily damaged. Some of that damage occurs as a result of natural processes, but the majority of it is caused by free radicals that mutate, or alter, DNA's original, perfect code. Eventually, if there is enough mutation, the instructions and information encoded within the DNA become so distorted that it can no longer send healthy operating instructions to your cells.

Disease is the result.

Experts concur that upward of 90 percent of all cancers, as well as heart disease and virtually all other degenerative disease, are the result of mutated DNA. Because of this, antioxidant-rich, free-radical-fighting phytonutrients are now considered to be on the cutting edge of disease prevention and reversal.

THE PHYTONUTRIENTS

Carotenoids

Carotenoids, the first of the phytonutrient families, all share the red and yellow pigments in carrots, tomatoes, and other fruits and vegetables. To date, more than 600 different carotenoids have been identified, among them *alpha, gamma, lutein,* and *zeaxanthan,* as well as the family's most prized members, *beta carotene* and *lycopene.*

Beta-carotene, most commonly found in apricots, cantaloupe, carrots, sweet potatoes, winter squash, and yams, has been found to lower the risk of a variety of cancers. Recent studies have found that those who had the highest amounts of beta carotene in their diet had a significantly lower risk of death from cancer.

Lycopene, most abundantly found in cooked tomatoes, is a powerful antioxidant. A Harvard study of 48,000 men found that those who ate ten half-cup servings of cooked tomatoes cut their risk of prostate cancer by 48 percent. Evaluating the prostate tissue of twenty-five men, researchers at Dana Farber Cancer Institute and Harvard Medical School also determined that tomato consumption was linked with a lowered incidence of prostate cancer.[1]

Lycopene has also been implicated in reductions in the risk of colon, rectal, and stomach cancers. It is important to note that cooking tomatoes greatly increases the availability of lycopene.

Other studies have confirmed that various carotenoids in leafy green vegetables, such as broccoli, kale, and spinach, significantly lower the risk of macular degeneration—the leading cause of eye disease in people older than fifty.

The most potent sources of carotenoids are broccoli, carrots, greens, and tomatoes. *The absorption of these carotenoids is enhanced by eating some fatty acids with them, such as olive oil.*

Flavonoids

Flavonoids, the second family of phytonutrients, include *anthocyanins, hesperidin, quercetin,* and *rutin.* Flavonoids are found most abundantly in apples, apricots, berries, endive, kale, onions, purple grapes, and red wine. Along with flavonoid's antioxidant properties, they also act as powerful heart protectors that help thin the blood, protecting against the formation of blood clots.

Recent laboratory studies have established that the flavonoids in red wine could, in some cases, prevent up to 100 percent of LDL (bad) blood cholesterol from oxidizing, and thus from clotting. Among other studies, flavonoids have been found to halt the progression of colon tumors in animals, lower the risk of stomach cancers, and reduce brain dysfunction and memory loss.

Monoterpenes

Monoterpene, the third family of phytonutrients, is found in cherries and citrus fruits and includes such compounds as *limonene,* found most abundantly in citrus oils and peels. Monoterpenes appear to have a special ability to fight the formation of cancerous tumors.

Recent university medical studies have established that laboratory animals given a limited diet of *limonene* showed a significant reduction in cancerous tumors. Elsewhere, researchers have established that limonene consistently encouraged cancer cells to self-destruct. Other studies have consistently shown that limonene increases the activity of proteins that eliminate estradiol—a hormone linked to breast cancer.

Perillyl alcohol is another monoterpene found in such plants as lavender and citrus fruits that has garnered attention in recent years. It has consistently demonstrated the ability to check cancers of the breast, lungs, stomach, liver, pancreas, and skin.

Polyphenolic Compounds

This fourth group of phytonutrients includes *catechins, curcumin,* and *ellagic acid.* Polyphenols are found most abundantly in green and black teas, all berries, olive oil, turmeric, most vegetables, and whole grains. Polyphenols have demonstrated profound anti-cancer effects, and researchers have established that ellagic acid reduces free radicals and detoxifies carcinogens. Meanwhile, other scientists are finding that the ellagic acid in olive oil provides powerful protection against free-radical damage, protecting both the arteries and breasts and lowering the risk of female breast cancers by as much as 25 percent.

Indoles and Isothiocyanates

The fifth group of phytonutrients includes *indole 3 carbinol* (13Cs) and *sulforaphane.* They are most abundantly found in broccoli, Brussels sprouts, cabbage, cauliflower, and mustard greens.

Scientists have discovered that 13Cs work as agents that sweep up excess harmful estrogens before they can contribute to cancer-cell development, while increasing levels of healthy faux-estrogens. A variety of population studies have shown 13Cs to be useful as protective agents against breast, cervical, colon, and prostate cancers.

Many oncology researchers are concluding that sulforaphan triggers the release of enzymes that rid the body of toxins, reducing the risk of free-radical damage and cancer.

Allylic Sulfides

The sixth group of phytonutrients are most abundantly found in garlic and onions. Among them are the compounds *diallyl disulfide* (DADS) and *diallyl trisulfide.*

In one recent study, men with elevated cholesterol were given a garlic extract rich in allylic sulfides. Many of them had as much as a 60 percent decrease in their platelet counts. Many similar studies are continually finding these compounds to be effective blood thinners, thus reducing the risk of heart disease.

Substances in garlic have been shown to slow the development of prostate cancer cells, and studies also suggest that certain of its active ingredients may also lower cholesterol, bring down high blood pressure, boost the immune system, and block carcinogens in foods eaten with garlic.[1]

Isoflavones

The seventh group of phytonutrients contain the currently popular *genistein* and *daidzein,* which are found abundantly in soybeans and their products, as well as in chick peas, kidney beans, and lentils.

Among the most powerful actions of isoflavones is the ability to act as regulators of hormones. Currently, many American women are using soy products and other isoflavone-containing foods to help mitigate the unpleasant effects of menopause and pre-menopause. Isoflavones help prevent harmful estrogens from attaching to cell receptors by attaching to the receptors themselves, thus blocking the action of the harmful estrogens, such as cancer-causing 16 alpha hydroxy esterone. In study after study, documented evidence shows that isoflavones are clearly reducing the risk of breast cancers. Isoflavones are also particularly good at lowering LDL cholesterol.

Saponins

Saponins, the eighth group of phytonutrients, are found in most beans and vegetables, some whole grains, and herbs. The most common sources are oats, peas, soybeans, and ginseng. Saponins help remove mucus from the lungs and stomach. They also provide anti-inflammatory support for the arteries and can help balance hormones, the metabolism, and mood swings. Recent studies have shown that saponins help lower LDL (bad cholesterol) levels, support bone health, work against certain cancers, and strengthen the immune system.

Lignans

Lignans, the ninth phytonutrient group, are plant estrogens that possess either estrogenic or anti-estrogenic properties. They provide immune-enhancing antioxidant activity. A number of studies have reported a direct correlation between high levels of lignans in the diet and reduced risks for breast, ovarian, and prostate cancer, heart disease, and osteoporosis. The most common sources of lignans are apricots, broccoli, cashew nuts, flaxseeds, kale, sesame seeds, strawberries, sunflower seeds, and all whole grain products.

Studies have shown that, after three months of eating an ounce and a half of soy flour daily, women had significantly fewer hot flashes. And several studies have documented that Japanese women, who traditionally eat soy regularly, have one of the lowest incidences of breast cancer in the world.

One of the more powerful cancer-preventive antioxidants in soy is genistein, which is thirty times higher in soy than in meat-based diets. This antioxidant has been shown in vitro to inhibit angiogenesis (blood-vessel growth), an important factor in ceasing cancer-cell growth.

Researchers have also proven that genistein regulates the cancer-suppressor gene P21, which works in tandem with the P53 gene in regulating cancer-cell growth.

A number of controlled studies continue to show that soy has an effective cancer-preventive effect on premenopausal women. One Australian study measured five different phytoestrogens and showed that women with the highest levels of phytoestrogens had a four-fold decrease in the risk for breast cancer.

In May 2008, scientists at Hanyang University in Korea found that when compared to the lowest soy users, premenopausal women who used the highest amount of soy had a 61 percent lower risk for breast cancer. For post-menopausal women, the risks were 78 percent lower for the highest soy users.

MY TOP TWENTY-FIVE PHYTONUTRIENT-RICH SUPER-FOODS

Foods have wondrous healing properties that science is just beginning to uncover. Vegetables and fruits, in particular, are powerful healers. Make use of them and help yourself to Nature's offerings by using this as one of your guides.

FOOD	PHYTONUTRIENT
1. Tomatoes	Carotenoids
2. Apricots	Carotenoids, flavonoids
3. Chicory	Carotenoids
4. Brussels sprouts	Indoles, isothiocyanates
5. Cabbage	Indoles, isothiocyanates
6. Broccoli	Carotenoids, indoles, isothiocyanates
7. Sweet potatoes, yams	Carotenoids
8. Blueberries	Flavonoids, polyphenols

9. Purple grapes	Flavonoids, polyphenols
10. Red wine	Flavonoids, polyphenols
11. Olive oil (*cold, first pressed, extra virgin*)	Polyphenols
12. Granny Smith Apples	Flavonoids
13. Onions	Allyl sulfides
14. Garlic	Allyl sulfides
15. Lemons	Monoterpenes
16. Oranges	Monoterpenes, flavonoids
17. Cherries	Monoterpenes
18. Turmeric	Polyphenols
19. Black pepper	Polyphenols
20. Tofu	Isoflavonoids
21. Black beans	Isoflavonoids
22. Oatmeal	Tocotrienols
23. Green tea	Polyphenols
24. Flaxseeds	Lignans
25. Strawberries	Polyphenols

Supplementing the Fight Against Disease

Vitamins, Minerals, and Other Natural Medicines

Americans take more than 3 billion nutritional supplements every day. Do It Yourself (or DIY) Health, as it's sometimes called, is nothing short of a millennial phenomenon.

According to a March 13, 2009, Nielsen study, 56 percent of American consumers currently use vitamins and dietary supplements, with 44 percent of these saying they use them daily.[1]

The net amount spent on the top-performing dietary supplements in the U.S. is estimated to be $24–25 billion per year, with some experts saying a more accurate estimate is likely to be in the $30–40 billion range. Total U.S. sales just for vitamins alone reached $7.4 billion in 2007. The top five vitamins sold were multivitamins, B-complex, C, D, and E.

During that same period, mineral sales reached $1.8 billion. The top five minerals sold were calcium, chromium, iron, magnesium, and potassium. Herbal and botanical sales hit $4.5 billion. The top five herbals and botanicals sold were garlic, green tea, mangosteen juice, noni juice, and saw palmetto.

In 2009, global nutriceutical sales were projected to reach $187 billion by 2010, buoyed by rising sales in China and India. With such large numbers of people taking natural compounds, it is obvious that many want to prevent illness and disease and enhance health in a natural way.

Making the correct decisions about which supplements to take is very important. In most cases, people read about particular supplements and then determine which ones they think would be good for them. In some cases, they visit a physician, or a nutritionist, or a natural health practitioner who makes certain suggestions. And while this may help you make better choices, it is still a shotgun approach that fails to consider your body chemistry, your constitution, and your lifestyle—in other words, *the whole person.*

For supplements to be their most effective, they need to be tailored to your bio-individuality. Therefore, it's best to be guided in your choices by a system that determines your unique constitutional and/or chemical needs. As I've said in earlier chapters, there are several effective techniques a practitioner can use to test your tolerances and needs for individual substances. The Chinese constitutional types system is one such method that can be very helpful.

HAIR ANALYSIS

Another strictly Western technique that uses a purely scientific method for determining bio-individuality is called TMA, or trace mineral analysis. TMA measures your body's mineral levels to get a picture of your present chemistry. Sometimes referred to as hair analysis (because hair is the substance tested), TMA is, in my opinion, by far the most useful clinical tool for assessing which nutritional supplements a person needs at a particular time.

The process is simple, accessible, and very inexpensive. Approximately one tablespoon of hair (200–500 mg) is taken (preferably from the nape of the neck). This sample is then sent off to a TMA laboratory where it is exposed to multiple acids and high temperatures that break down the hair, making the keratin (protein) contained in the third inner layer of the hair available for analysis. The minerals found in the keratin are then measured in quantities 1,000 times larger than the mineral concentrations measured in blood tests. The hair is analyzed using a highly sophisticated process called *atomic absorption spectroscopy*, which measures the hair's mineral concentrations. The minerals are measured in parts per million and printed on a graph. I've interpreted tens of thousands of TMA samples over the years and have found them to be remarkably accurate, useful indicators of overall metabolic patterns in the body.

Blood analysis gives a *poor* reflection of the body's overall nutritional levels. This is partly because the blood is such a vital transportation highway that the hypothalamus does everything it can to maintain the blood's biochemical equilibrium at all costs. That is to say, all possible essential nutrients are directed first to the blood and may be deficient in the rest of the body.

Hair (protein) is a much more accurate indicator of the true picture of a person's biochemistry and resulting biochemical needs. While I know there has been some debate over the years about the efficacy of TMA, I feel very strongly that it is an excellent indicator of individual nutritional needs. In order for this test to be useful and accurate, however, it is crucial that a high-quality laboratory be used, along with an experienced practitioner who can correctly interpret the results.

INTERPRETATIONS OF A HAIR ANALYSIS CHART

When interpreting a hair analysis chart, even before I look at the nutrient mineral levels on the front page, I check the significant mineral ratios. (*See* the sample chart on the following page.)

In the lab format, the first significant ratio is CA:MG (calcium to magnesium), which has a norm of 7:1. The second ratio CA:P (calcium to phosphorous), has a norm of 2.6:1. Third, there is MG:K (magnesium to potassium), which has a norm of 2.4:1. The fourth ratio, NA:K (sodium to potassium), has a norm of 2.4:1. The fifth ratio, ZN:CU (zinc to copper), has a norm of 8:1. The sixth ratio is ZN:CD (zinc to cadmium), which has a norm of 800:1.

These are all extremely significant markers of the metabolic chem - istries in the body. For example, the second and third ratios, calcium to phosphorous and magnesium to potassium, are both metabolic markers for the thyroid gland. They tell whether or not the gland is operating at its most efficient energy level. The fourth ratio, sodium to potassium,

Elements Regarded As Toxic

TOXIC ELEMENTS	PATIENT LEVEL (parts per million)			► HIGH
Aluminum	1	**		
Antimony	0.100	*********	.17	
Arsenic	0.090	*********	.15	
Beryllium	0.010	*****	.03	
Bismuth	<dl .001		.01	
Cadmium	0.300	**************	.25 *	
Lead	8.0	*************** .5	*********	
Mercury	2.90	************* 1.5	************	
Nickel	0.20	****	.17	
Platinum	0.001	*	.03	
Silver	0.10	****	0.4	
Thallium	<dl .001		.05	
Thorium	0.002	***	.01	
Tin	0.1	**	0.8	
Uranium	0.230	*************	.2 ***	

SAMPLE SIZE:	0.15 g
SAMPLE TYPE:	head hair
DATE SAMPLED:	01/01/1995
DATE IN:	01/01/95
DATE OUT:	01/31/95 R
OFFICE CODE:	2-2
	ICP-MS analyzed
RACE:	caucasian
HAIR COLOR:	gray
HAIR PREPS:	
SHAMPOO:	glycerin soap

Ratios

	PATIENT RATIO	EXPECTED RANGE	
CA/MG	18.7	5-	15
CA/P	0.8	2.6-	6.1
MG/K	0.1	1.8-	5.0
NA/K	1.4	1.8-	4.0
ZN/CU	13.9	4-	12
ZN/CD	323	>800	

TOTAL TOXIC REPRESENTATION **

Elements Regarded As Nutrients

NUTRIENT ELEMENT	PATIENT LEVEL (parts per million)	LOW ◆	REFERENCE RANGE	● HIGH	NUMERICAL VALUE OF REFERENCE ◆ RANGE ●
Calcium	112	*********************			280- 600
Magnesium	6	**********************			30- 75
Sodium	129		**************		20- 90
Potassium	77		*****************		9- 40
Copper	7	*****************			11- 28
Zinc	97	*****************			125- 155
Iron	8		******		5- 14
Manganese	0.16	*****************			0.30- 0.75
Chromium	0.44	***************			0.80- 1.25
Cobalt	<dl .001	*****************			0.020- 0.045
Vanadium	0.010	***************			0.009- 0.080
Molybdenum	0.070		**********		0.030- 0.080
Boron	1.80		**		0.80- 2.80
Iodine	0.1	*****************			0.3- 1.2
Lithium	0.020	*****************			0.050- 0.120
Phosphorus	134	****************			144- 204
Selenium	0.290	*****************			0.950- 1.700
Strontium	0.36	****************			0.50- 4.80
Sulfur	+1000	*****************			48000- 52500

Other Elements

ELEMENT	PATIENT LEVELS	EXPECTED RANGE	ONE STANDARD DEVIATION HIGH →	TWO STANDARD DEVIATIONS HIGH →
Barium	0.21	0.40- 2.50		
Germanium	0.003	0.003- 0.028		
Rubidium	<dl .001	0.020- 0.150		
Titanium	0.440	0.100- 0.700 ***		
Zirconium	0.300	0.020- 0.530 ***		

COMMENTS:

Hair analysis chart.

reflects the energy output of the adrenal cortex—the outer layer of the adrenal gland.

The ratio of calcium to potassium is not specifically listed in this chart as every lab displays a slightly different profile. The ratio of calcium to potassium, however, is a very important marker for the metabolic functioning of the thyroid. If the ratio of calcium to potassium is extremely high, it suggests a hypothyroid (low thyroid) state. A low ratio of calcium to potassium often reveals an overactive thyroid tendency. This is usually something that happens as a result of the sodium to magnesium ratio being extremely low. When sodium is very low in relation to magnesium, it indicates that the person's stress levels are too high, the adaptability to stress has been very poor, and the emotional, mental, or physical stress is overwhelming the body's chemistry and exhausting the adrenal medulla (the innermost portion of the adrenal gland). Once the adrenal glands have become exhausted, they demand emergency support from the thyroid gland, which then becomes exhausted as well.

The fifth significant ratio, zinc to copper, is a very good indicator for progesterone and testosterone, whereas the first ratio, calcium to magnesium, is a good indicator for estrogens and androgens. Finally, the ratio of iron to copper (not listed here, as each lab chooses to list different significant ratios) also reflects the working of the adrenal cortex.

So the ratios of sodium to potassium, sodium to magnesium, and iron to copper are the primary adrenal markers. I look very carefully at these in relation to the ratios of calcium to potassium (thyroid indicators) because when the adrenal glands become exhausted and the thyroid is pressed into service excessively it becomes exhausted too. This condition also decreases the body's ability to assimilate calcium. In many women with developing osteoporosis, the adrenal glands lie at the core of the problem. And simply putting such women on calcium supplements can create a host of additional problems. In most cases, the adrenal and thyroid glands need to be supported before the body can make safe and efficient use of the calcium supplements.

The nutrient mineral analysis chart shows the levels for 19 nutrient minerals, beginning with Ca, or calcium. The chart shows the normal reference range of each mineral as indicated by the pale, almost white horizontal (mean) strip in the center of the reference range and the range numbers at the far right. For example, calcium has a normal reference range of 280–600 ppm.

Above the top of the Nutrient mineral graph are the indicators for 15 toxic minerals. The levels for aluminum, arsenic, beryllium, cadmium, mercury, lead, etc., should in effect be zero, or as low as possible. Any indicators that these minerals are in the body is unfavorable and should be immediately addressed.

SUPPLEMENTS FOR BALANCING THE WHOLE PERSON

The following section contains a listing of the supplements that are most commonly recommended to balance out the vast majority of TMA results I have interpreted.

Vitamin A

I use vitamin A for exceptionally low or high calcium levels because it's an excellent calcium balancer. In helping the body assimilate calcium, it prevents excess quantities from depositing in the kidneys. I recommend that those with low calcium levels take 10,000 IU of oil-based vitamin A, along with 400 IU of vitamin D, every day.

Vitamin B_1

I use vitamin B_1 for exceptionally high or low adrenal ratio markers. Extremely high or low sodium to magnesium, sodium to potassium, or iron to copper ratios tell me the adrenal glands are working too hard or have exhausted themselves completely. In these cases, I will recommend high doses of vitamin B_1, also called thiamin, in a twice daily dosage of 100 mg with meals.

Vitamin B_2

Vitamin B_2 lowers the toxic mineral mercury, and I also use it to lower elevated boron. High levels of mercury and/or boron indicate that the kidneys are inflamed and are having a difficult time filtering proteins and cleaning themselves of endotoxins. When boron is elevated, it indicates a deficiency of vitamin B_2. In these cases, I recommend high doses of B_2: 100 mg twice a day with meals. When mercury is elevated, I recommend 200 mg of B_2 with meals three times daily.

Vitamin B_5

Also known as pantothenic acid, vitamin B_5 is needed whenever the ratios of sodium to potassium, sodium to magnesium, and iron to copper are out of balance. When the adrenal glands are overstressed, as indicated by these unbalanced ratios, I recommend 100 mg of B₅ twice a day with meals to strengthen the adrenals. High sodium to potassium ratios also indicates that adrenal stress has exhausted the cardiovascular system. The higher that ratio goes, the greater the cardiovascular stress. Vitamin B₅ reduces sodium and potassium, taking the burden off of the adrenal glands and the cardiovascular system.

Vitamin B₆

Also called pyridoxine hydrochloride, vitamin B₆ reduces high copper levels that build up in bile ducts, brain tissue, and liver tissue. This buildup accompanies inflammatory viruses and excessively high estrogen levels. High copper levels have also been linked to numerous health problems, such as certain cancers in women, chronic retroviruses, gallbladder disease, and inflammatory disease, including rheumatoid arthritis. I recommend 100 mg twice a day with meals.

Vitamin C

I like to use ascorbate (specifically vitamin C) to neutralize the effects of toxic minerals and endotoxins in the liver and kidneys. Because of its antioxidant properties, it's also a good immune enhancer. I recommend 3,000 mg (3 gm) per day.

Vitamin D

I suggest vitamin D whenever calcium levels are extremely low. I recommend doses of 400 IU per day, along with vitamin A, to enhance calcium metabolism.

Vitamin E

Vitamin E works well in conjunction with vitamins B₁ and B₅ for adrenal support. Whenever the ratios of sodium to potassium, sodium to magnesium, and iron to copper are out of balance, elevated, or dramatically depleted, it means that the adrenal glands are working overtime stressing the cardiovascular system. Vitamin E is very good at lowering the excess stores of tissue sodium and potassium, taking the burden off the adrenal glands and the heart. I recommend taking 400 IU per day of the d-alpha form of vitamin E.

Calcium

I recommend calcium whenever I see that the TMA chart indicates extremely low calcium levels. I also sometimes recommend calcium when the chart shows extremely high calcium levels. This may sound contradictory, but often when calcium tissue levels are high, it indicates that calcium is not circulating in the blood, but is instead sedimenting (settling) into the tissues because of highly acidic blood. Calcium threonate alkalizes the blood and absorbs very efficiently rather than depositing itself as stones. Thus, I prefer the calcium threonate form in a dose of 1,000 mg per day, taken in the same pill together with 500 mg of magnesium taureate.

Magnesium

Along with calcium, magnesium is very important for alkalizing the blood and tissues, supporting the adrenal glands, and tranquilizing the nervous system when stress levels are high. Magnesium can also help with insomnia. (*See* dose recommendations for calcium in this list.)

Zinc

I prefer zinc gluconate taken in conjunction with vitamin B_6 to lower elevated copper levels. I suggest a dosage of 50 mg per day.

Iron

When a mineral is low in the TMA, it usually indicates that the individual is not able to assimilate the particular nutrient efficiently. Because of this, it isn't simply a matter of giving the nutrient, but also making sure it can be assimilated. Iron bisglycinate is generally referred to as gentle iron because it's most easily assimilated and tends not to cause constipation. I recommend 30–50 mg of iron bisglycinate per day with a meal. As another option, I also often recommend two tsp. of Floravital per day.

Chromium GTF (Glucose Tolerance Factor)

Low levels of chromium indicate to me that blood sugar is not being properly managed by the body and that insulin levels are either very high or low. This means that the individual most likely needs fewer high-starch carbohydrates and should be eating more protein and low-starch carbohydrates. I recommend 200 mg taken at mealtime once a day. If the chromium levels are lower than .01 mg in the chart, I suggest taking it twice a day.

Selenium

Selenium is another very important indicator for thyroid. Whenever I see a TMA chart with extremely high calcium to potassium ratios and/or extremely high calcium to phosphorous ratios, I look at the selenium because it reflects the activity of a thyroid hormone called T_3, the most activating thyroid hormone. If I find low selenium, it suggests the likelihood of a low thyroid condition. This situation is a good example of a case in which blood tests alone are particularly poor indicators of thyroid function. The best indicators are blood combined with TMA and basal temperature readings. (Underarm temperature should be 97.8.)

Multi-Enzymes

When I see elevated calcium, it indicates to me that calcium isn't being efficiently digested or assimilated, but is, instead, being stored in such places as the kidneys and arteries. Excess calcium can contribute to the formation of kidney stones and arterial blockages. Enzymes, specifically hydrochloric acid (available in multi-enzymes), are largely responsible for digesting calcium. Take one with each of three meals a day.

Pectin

I suggest pectin whenever I see elevated levels of aluminum, arsenic, beryllium, cadmium, lead, or mercury in the toxic mineral chart. Pectin binds with these toxic minerals to help carry them out of the body. Pectin should be taken in a dosage of two 250 mg tablets before bedtime so it does not bind with other supplements or food nutrients.

Raw Thyroid Tablets and Raw Adrenal Tablets

These tablets are useful when imbalances are detected in the adrenal ratios of sodium to potassium, sodium to magnesium, and iron to copper in relation to the thyroid ratios of calcium to phosphorus and calcium to potassium. These tablets contain ribonucleic acid that can bond with cellular codes so that bovine sources from which the tablets are made will actually strengthen the corresponding human organs. Once available only by injection in European health spas, these bio-regulating supplements are now available in freeze-dried tablet form. I recommend taking 150–200 mg tablets of raw thyroid and raw adrenal (from bovine sources fed on organic foods) with meals twice a day.

L-Tyrosine

The amino acid L-tyrosine is a direct precursor of both adrenal and thyroid hormones, and its use is indicated when I see imbalances in the ratios of calcium to phosphorus, calcium to potassium, and sodium to magnesium. It helps control anxiety, appetite, and depression. I recommend 500 mg taken once a day between meals.

Ciwugia

Also known as wild Siberian ginseng, research has shown that ciwugia increases stamina and supports adrenal and thyroid function. I recommend taking two 400 mg tablets in the morning and afternoon on an empty stomach.

17

The Spirit Ill at Ease

How is your spirit ill at ease? What's troubling you? What are the patterns at work in your life and how did they begin? These are the first and most important questions I ask every patient I see.

Regardless of your physical condition, I know that in order to heal, you must be whole, and that to be whole, your mind, body, and heart must be integrated and nurtured. If you're not integrated, if you disregard your inner *spirit self,* you will become dissociated, fragmented, and cut off from the life-energy—and healing—source of your being.

I believe that the disintegration I see in so many people has come about as a result of this culture's focus on the external world. Where the ancestors once lived a more integrated mind/body/spirit existence, today's culture has become almost exclusively focused on the physical/material/external. This materialistic bias has become the foremost mind-shaper, and popular culture has convinced everyone that they are little more than personality-driven bodies. The unmistakable message that comes through is that if you fail to conform to the ideal materialistic image of who you should be, you are somehow incomplete. Having been conditioned by this one pervasive message, that you are not good enough as you are, you believe you must attain something outside yourself in order to be complete. But the fact is, who you are does *not* depend upon what you have. Nor does ignoring any of the elements of self—be it mind, body, or spirit—help you to achieve a peaceful, healthy, stress-free way of life.

Chinese medicine is rooted in the ancient Chinese belief that everyone's spirit ingests everything it sees, hears, smells, thinks, tastes, and feels, and that everyone is fed and shaped by these influences.

If you bombard your senses with an endless barrage of pop culture's meaningless sex, violence, and greed, if you burden your biological system with toxins and intolerable foods, you risk becoming unhealthy in every sense of the word.

The truth that people are spiritual begins the conflict between the materialism practiced and the unfulfilled needs of the spirit, and this creates chaos, which results in disintegration, a sense of separation from other people, self-contempt, and ultimately . . . dis-ease. Because the spirit is traumatized by disintegration, it is actually creating bodily disease.

When I look into the hearts and minds of so many whom I treat each day, I see a growing mistrust in the world's social systems, its governmental authorities, and its institutions. Where strength and integrity were once perceived, there is now the assumption of weakness and falsehood. A socio-cultural phase of external disintegration has come to exist, typified by the breakdown of institutions, including business, education, government, and social, even the family itself, and the onset of cynicism, fear, and uncertainty. In the process, there is also a disintegration that takes place between races, genders, and age groups.

The only way to begin to reverse this process is through the individual. Regardless of present patterns in the external world, the human instinct to fulfill the body/mind/spirit must be integrated. There was a time when you could almost always count on the love, trust, and integral support of the external world: mother, father, family, and society. This is no longer necessarily so. Thus the need to adapt to circumstances and turn inward for the support, trust, and love necessary to thrive and prosper. If it truly takes a village to raise a child, then everyone needs to create that village within the *self*.

Every Chinese taoist was taught both fishing and farming. When there was no wind to propel their sailboats, they ate from their vegetable gardens. When the gardens were damaged by drought or flood, they set sail to harvest fish from the sea. In other words, they adapted themselves to fit the circumstances of their lives, and they did so in a way that promoted harmony within their *self*.

Now is the time for everyone to learn the art of adaptation between the universal poles of yin and yang, mind and body, spirit and ego. Now is the time for everyone to find integration, healing, and wholeness within themselves, to cultivate their own healing spirit.

The best way to do this is to integrate all the parts: the right brain with the left, the past with the present, intuition with logic, emotions with intellect, the vulnerable child self with the powerful parent self. In this way, it is possible to become truly aware of these polarities and learn to honor each of them. Working toward self-integration will serve to reclaim the natural wholeness that holds the key to healing. Everyone deserves to be whole, to heal, and to be completed in love. But it must first be acknowledged that completed love can only be engaged within an unconditional, autonomous, integrated human being.

The following is a script for a guided visualization that is aimed at helping you integrate mind and heart. Please record it for yourself. In this way you'll be listening to your voice guiding you. Listen to it frequently. I've used this program to help literally thousands of people cultivate a spirit of self-integration. It begins with a brief relaxation exercise. For best results, wear comfortable, loose-fitting clothing and find a time when you will not be disturbed as you do the exercise.

INTEGRATION VISUALIZATION

Relax. Take a slow, deep breath through your nose as you fill your lungs. Hold the breath, then release it through your mouth. Once again, take a slow, deep breath through your nose, hold the breath, and release it through your mouth. Now, finally, take a third deep breath through your nose, hold, then release through your mouth.

As you relax, in your mind's eye picture your left foot and your left leg. Feel them both. Tense all the muscles in your left foot and your left leg. Tighten them as much as you can. Now, take a deep breath through your nose as you continue to tense your left leg and foot. Now, at the count of three, simultaneously release both your breath and the tension you are holding in your muscles. One . . . two . . . three . . . now completely release your breath and the tension.

Next, focus your mind's eye and your attention on your right foot and your right leg as you breathe in through your nose. Tense all the muscles in you right foot and right leg as tightly as you can. Hold and intensify that tension for a moment. (Pause) Now, at the count of three, release your breath and release the tension and stress in your right foot and right leg. One . . . two . . . three . . . release your breath and the tension.

Now, focus your mind's eye and your attention on your left arm and hand as you breathe in. Tense all the muscles in your left arm and hand as tightly as you can. Hold and intensify that tension for a moment. (Pause) Now, at the count of three, release your breath and release the tension and stress in your left arm and hand. One . . . two . . . three . . . release your breath and the tension.

Next, focus your mind's eye and your attention on your right hand and arm as you breathe in through your nose. Tense all the muscles in your right hand and arm as tightly as you can. Hold and intensify that tension for a moment. (Pause) Now, at the count of three, release your breath, and release the tension and stress in your right hand and arm. One . . . two . . . three . . . release your breath and the tension.

Now, picture in your mind's eye your mid-torso, your stomach, your abdomen, your lower back, your upper back. Tense your abdominal muscles, your back muscles, your pectoral (chest) muscles, and prepare to sweep the stress away from all these muscles and vital organs simultaneously with the release of your breath. Once you're tensed up, take a deep breath through your nose, hold that breath, tense your body even more, then, at the count of three, release your breath and the tension. One . . . two . . . three . . . release your breath and the tension.

Now, in your mind's eye, picture your face, the top of your head, the sides and back of your head. Tighten up all your facial muscles. In a moment, you are going to release all the stress from your mind and your thoughts. Take a deep breath in through your nose. (Pause) At the count of three, release all your stresses and tensions as you breathe out through your mouth. One . . . two . . . three . . . release all breath and tension.

At this point, you feel very deeply relaxed. You are very aware of your entire being. You are in a deep, deep state of tranquil peace and relaxation. And now, as you rest peacefully, imagine that you are floating up toward a soft, puffy cloud. (Pause) You are traveling light as a feather, ascending slowly to that cloud. (Pause) You reach the cloud, and you settle yourself into it, lying restfully on that soft, comfortable cloud. The cloud is your transportation through time. It will carry you back into the past, to a time in your childhood. Relax as you travel.

You slowly arrive at your destination. And as you do, it's time to very slowly put your feet and legs over the edge of the cloud and let yourself float slowly down to Earth, still as light as a feather. You notice familiar surroundings and familiar faces. You see your home, your neighborhood, your street. You see friends and family. As you continue to look around, you touch down at last and see your child self. She or he is whatever image you first picture in your mind. Regardless of whether or not your childhood memories are positive or negative, you are completely secure in your present state and you are happy to have this reunion with the spirit of your child self. As you see, feel, and flow from your heart, your senses are drawn first to your child's natural innocence, which radiates from his or her eyes and heart.

Slowly, you approach your child self with all your natural instincts of love and nurturance. The world you left behind only temporarily blinded you to these instincts to love and nurture unconditionally. Now, as you gaze into the eyes of your child self, your deep desire to forgive, to love, and to nurture unconditionally are welling up from deep within you. Take this time now to speak from the heart to your child self. Send your thoughts, communicate your love telepathically.

Take some moments to enjoy this reunion. (Pause) Bask in this unification between your present and your past, your peaceful mind and your loving heart, your power and your vulnerability. Hold your child self close to you as you open your hearts to each other. Both of you are sharing in this long-awaited moment of tenderness. (Pause)

Now, ask your child self to come into your heart, to spiritually meld with you. Integrate this child deep within yourself. Tell your child, "I want to love and care for you, nurture you, and take you back with me so you can become one with me unconditionally." (Pause) Then, slowly, let the spirit of your forgotten child self come into your heart. (Pause) You are rescuing that child with your attention and love. You are now giving your child self a long-awaited, loving home in your heart. (Pause) This marks the end of your dis-integrated life and the beginning of your integration. Feel the blending of your past with your present, your heart with your mind, your vulnerability with your strength. (Pause)

Together, you and your child self will rise up to the cloud that transported you here. Light as a feather, fully integrated, you both rise slowly to the top of the cloud. You rest atop the cloud, fully integrated and at peace. Your body, mind, and spirit are one. You are filled with an internal sense of compassion and an unconditional love such as you've never known before.

You are transported back through time and space, once again arriving in the present. As your cloud arrives and gently stops, you sit up and dangle your feet over the edge of the fluffy surface. Lightly, you float back to Earth, back into your daily life. But you enter your life as never before. Now all the care, all the love, all the support you've ever needed in your life is suddenly right there inside you, coming from deep within your own spirit. You know that from this time forward, you will always seek within yourself to fulfill your vital needs. You are no longer blind to the world's lie, and you are no longer victim to the world's false promise. You are fully integrated within.

Take a few minutes now to slowly return to the present moment. Do not rush off. It is important to reflect on what you have just done and, most important of all, on the person you are becoming.

I have always found this integration visualization exercise to have a profound healing impact. Maximum healing begins with whole-ism and true human whole-ism is rooted in the solidarity of the mind, heart, and spirit at peace within a happy body home.

In my work, I often use the metaphor that refers to the mind as the father, the heart as the mother, and the spirit as the child. They all live together within the home (body), and only when the father (mind) and the mother (heart) are truly married to each other is the child (spirit) safe to thrive and grow within a healthy home (body) environment. Through this metaphor, you can see that the physical health you seek so desperately truly begins with autonomous integral selfhood. Practice the visualization above and I think you will be able to cultivate love and trust within yourself. In the process, you will reintroduce your inner family to each other. The closer together the parts of your whole become, the closer you will be to knowing true and profound healing.

Questions and Answers

QUESTIONS RELATED TO WEIGHT LOSS

Q How can I lose weight safely and naturally, and keep it off?

A Each day, eat three half-cup servings of fresh, whole, raw fruit (not fruit juices) and three half-cup servings of fresh, whole, low-starch vegetables, such as asparagus, broccoli, cauliflower, celery, green beans, kale, salad greens, spinach, summer squash, and tomatoes. Eat no more than two half-cup servings daily of starch (breads, cereal, cookies, crackers, pasta, potatoes, and rice) daily. You must limit fat intake (oil) to two tbsp. per day and butter to two tsp. per day. The healthiest cooking oils are avocado oil, centrifuge coconut oil, cold-pressed extra virgin olive oil, grapeseed oil, and macadamia oil. These are the most heat-resistant and are the least inclined to unbalance existing ratios of essential fatty acids. Canola oil is favorably monounsaturated, but it is highly genetically modified. I suggest avoiding it.

Q Are there any natural food supplements that would naturally suppress my appetite?

A The amino acid L-phenylalanine 50 mg, one mid-morning and one mid-afternoon. Also, psyllium husk powder, one teaspoon before meals three times daily in 10 oz. of water.

Q Are there any food supplements that would naturally suppress my sugar cravings?

A The amino acid L-glutamine, 500 mg, one mid-morning and one mid-afternoon, and the mineral chromium GTF (glucose tolerance factor), 200 mcg, twice a day with food.

Q Which snack foods are both healthy and satisfying?

A Fresh fruit, almond nut butter spread blended with rice syrup, and dairy-free soy cream cheese. Occasionally, you can also have a dairy-free ice cream product made of rice cream.

Q Can hair analysis help me in my strategies to lose weight?

A Yes, hair analysis can help you better strategize for weight loss as it displays your mineral ratios of calcium to potassium, which indicates how efficiently, or inefficiently, your thyroid is burning calories. Furthermore, by taking the amino acid L-tyrosine, 1,000 mg a day on an empty stomach, you can help rebalance your errant metabolism as indicated by this hair analysis ratio.

Q Why are many over-the-counter weight-loss drugs potentially harmful for me?

A Weight-loss drugs not only artificially stimulate weight-loss mechanisms in the body, but in the heart and nervous systems as well, leading to elevated blood pressure and heart rate. In the long-term, they can exhaust an already depleted metabolism, further limiting the body's potential for weight loss.

Q What is the best form of exercise?

A Research says that a minimum of thirty minutes of brisk walking three times a week lowers virtually all health risk factors while optimizing energy metabolism and weight loss potential.

QUESTIONS RELATED TO MANAGING STRESS

Q How can unmanaged chronic stress speed up my aging process?

A The acid that builds up in your blood from chronic stress exhausts energy reserves at a far greater rate. In addition, the more stress hormones you secrete, the more you speed up cell death.

Q How does stress cause heart disease and cancer?

A Stress increases the body's productions of glandular hormones, which expedite the cellular loss of electrons. Once healthy cells lose their electrons, the probability of contracting cancer or heart disease is significantly increased.

Q How does unmanaged stress affect my appetite?

A Long-term stress increases the acidity of the body, which uses up vital nutrients more rapidly, thereby increasing the appetite.

Q What can I eat during periods of stress to reduce both my appetite and my stress levels?

A Increasing your intake of fruits and vegetables during periods of acute stress will help alkalize your blood. This will reduce your appetite and stress levels.

Q How can hair-mineral analysis help me in my strategies for fighting stress?

A The protein in your hair (keratin) is the best vehicle for determining the three key stress mineral ratios: sodium to potassium, sodium to magnesium, and iron to copper. These ratios are the keys to how your cells, vital organs, and glands are capable of managing stress. Hair-mineral analysis further shows how you can best support your body with diet and natural supplements during the recovery process.

Q When my body nutrients are out of balance, am I more
susceptible to the ravages of stress?

A Yes. However, using diagnostic and preventive means, such as hair-
mineral analysis, proper diet, and nutritional supplementation, can
significantly increase your adaptation response to stress.

Q What is the best natural way I can reduce stress quickly?

A Recent research suggests that the herb kava-kava root is an
extremely effective, safe, and over-the-counter way to reduce stress
quickly. Most studies seem to indicate that the average adult requires a
dose of kava-kava that provides a least 125 mg of the root's active ingre-
dient, kavalactones, in order to be effective. I recommend 125–150 mg
of kava-kava root along with a series of deep breathing exercises. Kava
kava should not be taken with any prescription pharmaceutical medications. There are rare but potential risk factors associated with the use of
kava kava. Elevated liver enzymes have been reported in twenty-five cases,
and one case of hepatitis has been reported to date.

QUESTIONS RELATED TO IMPROVING ENERGY

Q What foods will improve my energy?

A Increasing your intake of high-starch carbohydrates, such as brown
rice, fruits, potatoes, sweet potatoes, whole grain breads and pastas, whole grain cereals, and winter squash will generally improve your
energy as they readily convert into glucose, the body's high-octane fuel.

Q Are there any safe natural supplements that will improve
my energy?

A The best safe energy enhancers that I know are a Twin Labs amino-
acid product called *Glutamine Fuel* and wild Siberian ginseng. I

recommend 500–1,000 mg of Glutamine Fuel or 500–1,000 mg of wild Siberian ginseng capsules taken daily. Both are best absorbed on an empty stomach and should not be taken with prescription drugs.

Q How can hair-mineral analysis help me to increase my energy?

A The hair-mineral analysis ratio of calcium to magnesium is an important indicator of how efficiently your glands and organs are processing glucose, the body's fuel for energy. If calcium and magnesium tissue stores are in balance, and chromium and other mineral levels are low, you can increase your energy levels with 200 mcg of chromium GTF (glucose tolerance factor) twice per day with meals.

Q What can I do to conserve energy and relax my mind in the face of acute stress?

A Taking 500 mg magnesium chelate per day will generally relax the nervous system. In addition, you can take 50 mg of 5HTP (hydroxyl tryptophan), which is an amino acid, two times daily on an empty stomach. This will increase the brain's neurotransmitters that relax and refresh the mind and body.

QUESTION RELATED TO IMPROVING SEX DRIVE

Q Is there a natural way to improve sex drive and performance?

A The hair mineral analysis ratio between zinc and copper is a vital hormone marker that can reveal underlying sex drive and performance problems. When a problem exists, there is often a high copper to zinc ratio. Thus, 50 mg of zinc gluconate along with 200 mg of vitamin B_6 and 800 IU of d-alpha tocopherol E will, in time, improve these conditions.

Resources

Analytical Research Labs (ARL)
2225 W. Alice Avenue
Phoenix, Arizona 85021
Ph: (602) 995-1580 or (800) 528-4067
Website: www.arltma.com
A highly respected and experienced laboratory for hair-tissue mineral analysis that I have worked with over the years.

The Center for Food Safety (CFS)
660 Pennsylvania Ave, SE, #302
Washington DC 20003
Ph: (202) 547-9359,
Fax:(202) 547-9429
Email: office@centerforfoodsafety.org
Website: www.centerforfoodsafety.com
A non-profit public interest, environmental organization established for the purpose of challenging harmful food production technologies and promoting sustainable alternatives.

Institute for Responsible Technology
P.O. Box 469
Fairfield, Iowa 52556
Ph: 641.209.3604

Fax: 888-329-7000
Email: info@seedsofdeception.com
Website: www.seedsofdeception.com
Website for book of the same name by author Jeffrey Smith. It contains a non-GMO shopping list.

Linus Pauling Institute
Oregon State University
571 Weniger Hall
Corvallis, Oregon 97331-6512
Ph: 541-737-5075
Fax: 541-737-5077
Email: lpi@oregonstate.edu
Website: http://lpi.oregonstate.edu/
The Institute's website documents studies demonstrating that vitamin C lowers the risks for cardiovascular disease, stroke, hypertension, certain cancers, cataracts, and diabetes, and counteracts the ill effects of both lead poisoning and the common cold.

Micro Essential Laboratory, Inc.
4224 Avenue H
Brooklyn, New York 11210
Ph: 718-338-3618
Fax: 718-692-4491
Website: http://microessentiallab.com/
pH paper and pH strips for specialty testing, including urine.

Trace Elements Incorporated (TEI)
4502 Sunbelt Drive
Addison, Texas 75001
Ph: (800) 824-2314
Website: www.traceelements.com
This is another superior hair-tissue mineral analysis lab that I've worked with over the years and am currently using.

References

Chapter 2

1. Ni, H-C. *Entering The Tao—Master Ni's Teachings on Self-Cultivation.* Boston, MA: Shambhala Publications, 1997.

Chapter 3

1. Hu, FB, Stampfer, MJ, Manson, JE, et al. "Dietary Fat Intake and the Risk of Coronary Heart Disease in Women." *New England Journal of Medicine.* (337):1491–1499, Nov 20, 1997.

Chapter 14

1. Shelton, H. *Food Combining Made Easy.* Coplay, PA: Willow Publishing, 1982.

2. Smith, JM. *Seeds of Deception.* Fairfield, IA:Yes! Books, 2003.

Chapter 15

1. Yeager, S. and Eds. "New Foods for Healing—Capture the Powerful Cures of More than 100 Common Foods." *Prevention Magazine.* Emmaus, PA: Rodale Press, Inc. 1998.

Chapter 16

1.The Nielsen Company. "North America, Asia Lead Vitamin and Supplement Usage." Nielsen blog. www.nielsen.com. March 13, 2009.

Index

Quercetin, 192
Quinoa, 105, 106

Raspberries, 90
Raw adrenal tablets, 208
Raw kidney tablets, 146
Raw thyroid tablets, 208
Red clover, 118
Red Lentil Stew, 106
Relaxation, 155, 211–213
Respiration and respiratory diseases, 23,
    128, 130, 131
Rhemmannia, 147
Ribonucleic acid. 208
Rice, 122, 137, 149
Rice Pilaf with Almonds, 122
Rice pudding, 135
Rice syrup, 216
Roasted Chicken Breast, 152
Roasted Turkey Breast, 123
Root Vegetable Medley, 124
Rosemary, 151, 152
Rosemary Roasted Potatoes, 151
Rutin, 193
Rye berries, 105

S.O.D., 88
SAD. *See* Diet, Standard American (SAD).
Sadness, 61
Salads, 90, 93, 107–108, 109, 138
Salmon, 151
Salmon Kebobs, 151
Saponins, 196
Science, 9
Scrambled Tofu with Soy Links, 90
Seasons, 50–52, 58, 59, 60, 79, 95,
    111, 125, 141, 182
Seeds of Deception (Smith), 189–190
Selenium, 207
Self-identity and integration, 4–5,
    54–55, 209–214
Serotonin, 87
Sex drive, 217
Sheldrak, Rupert, 15

Shelton, Herbert M., 183
Shen Wung, 167
Shrimp, 106
Side effects, 16, 168
Sleep, 87, 115
Smith, Jeffrey, 189–190
Snacks, 216
Sodium, 205–206
Soft drinks, 182
Soups, 92, 107, 122–123, 138
Soy and soybeans, 35, 90, 91, 183, 189,
    195–196
Spirituality, 3–4, 7, 14, 209–214
Spleen, 58, 59, 60, 98, 113–114, 118
Spongia tosta, 132
Spring, 50, 58, 79
Squash, 122, 154
Squaw vine. *See* Black cohosh.
St. Johns wort, 45
Stamina, 117, 208
Starches, 36–39, 184, 217
Statins, 86
Stews, 106, 139
Stir-Fried Shrimp with Quinoa, 106
Stomach, 59, 60, 113
Strawberries, 90
Stress, 25, 119, 171–177, 203, 206,
    217–216
Stress response. *See* Fight or flight stress
    response.
Sugar, 33, 37, 117, 182, 216
Sulforphane, 195
Summer, 50, 51, 59, 95
Super Max EPA, 88
Super Oxide Dismutase. *See* S.O.D.
Supplements, 43, 199–208
Sweet potatoes, 154
Symptoms, 16–17, 19–20, 26

Ta'i ch'i, 155–164
Tam, Tom, 156
Tao, 14, 21
TCM. *See* Medicine, traditional Chinese
    (TCM).

About the Author

Mark Mincolla, Ph.D., is a nutritional and natural health therapist, energy healer, and medical intuitive who has studied extensively for many years with recognized Masters of Eastern Medicine and healing arts. Integrating ancient Chinese techniques with cutting-edge nutritional science, Mincolla centers his work on the bio-individuality of each patient he treats. In his private practice at Santi Holistic Healing in Cohasset, MA, through his frequent seminars and lectures, on his weekly television and radio shows that air in New England and are podcast nationally at markmincolla.com, as well as through the books he has authored, Mincolla has helped thousands of people in his three decades of practice.

The author graduated from Franklin Pierce College with a B.A. in psychology, received an M.A. in nutrition from Goddard College, and a Ph.D. in Health and Human Services from Columbia Pacific University. He and his wife Cecelia live in the south-shore suburbs of Boston. They have two sons, Nick and Lex, and a daughter Vanessea. The author can be contacted through his website at www.markmincolla.com.

www.ingramcontent.com/pod-product-compliance
Lightning Source LLC
Jackson TN
JSHW011359130125
77033JS00023B/743